Participatory Research in the Post-Normal Age

Leandro Luiz Giatti

Participatory Research in the Post-Normal Age

Unsustainability and Uncertainties to Rethink Paulo Freire's *Pedagogy of the Oppressed*

Springer

Leandro Luiz Giatti
School of Public Health
University of São Paulo
São Paulo, Brazil

ISBN 978-3-030-27923-3 ISBN 978-3-030-27924-0 (eBook)
https://doi.org/10.1007/978-3-030-27924-0

This Springer imprint is published by the registered company Springer Nature Switzerland AG
The registered company address is: Gewerbestrasse 11, 6330 Cham, Switzerland

When I learned how to prepare a pea soup, it seemed to be comfortable and fast. Fried bacon and onion, peas, potato, salt, and water, cooked for twenty minutes in a pressure cooker.
But when João cooked a pea soup for us, it took about three hours to be ready. That´s because, beyond making delicious and healthy food, he knew more and created much more. In rituals, we had great times of interaction, good coexistence, fun, and mutual learning among family and friends. The soup and any other culinary treasures were part of the outcomes within all of this.
This book is dedicated to João B Giatti, who as an uncle, a brother, and an amazing unforgettable friend, was wise.

Preface

There are three main reasons that I can point out for writing this book. The first is academic, to contribute to the contemporary development of participatory research, emphasizing new necessary understandings and fostering expansion of potentialities and applicabilities. The second is a political motivation, mainly considering that the decision on this kind of research is entirely associated with collaborative learning and acting in the real world to reduce neglected and emergent vulnerabilities. The last is a personal motivation to dialog with the very recent dynamics to reinforce reflections and pathways to this moment of superficiality and growth of radical and intolerant positions.

Towards academic inducement, the inspiration from Paulo Freire´s *Pedagogy of the Oppressed* is the starting point and the main thread for developing and rereading such a vital text on contemporary contexts and uncovered complexities. That is why the socio-ecological background suits the discussions, also because of the recognition of causal interdependencies that claim for hybrid knowledge and integrated actions. Such a stance imposes itself in the cross-scale problematization and searches for multistakeholder collaborative actions. Then, the dialogical process of interaction and intersubjectivity seem to be a powerful asset for including vulnerable and peripheric social groups into the sustainability and health debate—also, the characteristics of the "alive" processes of researching-learning present possible alternatives to encompass uncertainties.

In my conception, there is no possibility of searching for sustainability and better conditions of life and health without having cognitive justice and ecology of knowledge. Accordingly, multiple forms of engagement, reciprocal, and dialogical learning involving different social actors are at the core of compelling multilayered systems of interactions necessary to cope with the global scenarios of unsustainability. So, the role of reflexive practices in knowledge production can have new meanings and feasibility in such contexts and demands.

The political motivation is entirely intrinsic in that way, since the decision on proceeding with participatory research is political imperative, without forgetting the potential of scientific production. Effectively, knowledge production in participatory research presents itself as a democratic opening, because of the nature of learning collaboratively as acting on real societal concerns. The democratization of knowledge is also a central issue in the post-normal science criticism. Therefore, participatory research, in my view, complies with the paramount proposal of extending peer communities and making fairer relationships on the critical control of application and decision-making on scientific statements and innovation.

The third reason for me to present this book is the personal motivation that aligns with the staggering growth of societal fragmentations, intolerance, radicalisms, lack of reflexive interactions, and rejection on universal values like human rights, social justice, and ecological prudence. I cannot make a reliable panorama of such a spread and multi-factorial phenomena, but I have had a perception that the connectivity of the new virtual world has played a role in deepening changes in mindsets, as well as in dangerous unfolding. Also, these shifts have shown me a trend of hazardous alienation on issues that demand urgent actions like climate change and possible related consequences.

Somewhat, the ascension of radicalism and intolerance has demonstrated inconsequential and partial judgments, anti-science postures (like mistrust of vaccination), and moreover, aversion to critical dialog involving social actors, mainly those who have always been historically marginalized.

In Brazil, for example, people who affirm themselves as "liberal" are actively discouraging and depreciating the Freirean educational legacy, which is a world-renowned libertarian pedagogy. Indeed, it seems that they have the intent of being liberal in the economy but conservative in traditions, which calls attention for a worrying inclination on behalf of included social groups in keeping the traditional social order, maintaining a vast population group in social exclusion. Maybe for those with such aspirations, it seems to be convenient to restrain dialogical interaction and empowerment for vulnerable people. Anyhow, what has been occurring in the Brazilian context has similarities with international conjunctures. Thus, the reluctance in the liberation of the oppressed can be verified broadly disseminated, also resembling other times, like decades ago on the Cold War tensions.

For such contexts and struggles, other revolutionary theories must be developed to operate what would be the dialogical interactions to cope with the current global crisis of unsustainability and interrelated crises, in scenarios permeated by uncertainties and demanding urgent transitions. The challenging contemporary searches in that way also have to consider the burden of the transformations of communicative settings as the digital social networks, the rise of fear, misinformation, and misuse of science. Moreover, another foremost issue is that there is a need to reinforce reflection and broad engagement of stakeholders to critically control the employment of uncertain scientific statements to make decisions permeated by high stakes on unknown or neglected risks.

This book is conceived as a contribution to previous and still vigorous ideas reinterpreted in the contexts of unsustainability, risks, health iniquities, complexities, and uncertainties. Then, participatory research is considered as a possibility to foster interactions and necessary actions in the concrete reality for face-to-face engagement of distinguished stakeholders.

São Paulo, Brazil Leandro Luiz Giatti

Acknowledgments

To professors that have collaborated with joint reflections: Pedro Roberto Jacobi, Renata Ferraz de Toledo, Maria Cecilia Focesi Pelicioni, Aristides Almeida Rocha, Gabriela Marques Di Giulio, Rodolfo Andrade de Gouveia Vilela, Pedro Fernandes de Freitas, Nina Wallerstein, and Jutta Gutberlet. To researchers that have instigated ideas: Carolina Monteiro de Carvalho, Ricardo Agum, Carlos Tato Cortizo, Tania Mezzomo Keinert, Ana Maria Bedran Martins, Susanne Börner, Lira Luz Benites Lázaro, Alexandre Magno Barbosa, Rafael Buralli, and Sávio Stoco. To various students that arose interest and purposes, among them: Alberto Urbinatti, Simone Omori Honda, Rosicler Rodriguez, Mateus Amaral, Elizabeth Salinas Rebolledo, Juma Amanda Santos, Nadine Galbes, Rubens Landin, Amanda Silveira Carbone, Ana Cláudia Sanches Baptista, Aline Inácio Alves, and Camila Paulino. To FAPESP and São Paulo state society for funding my current research, mainly through the thematic project MacroAmb (proc.n.2015/03804-9, and proc.n. 2019/12804-3). To people from Iauaretê, Amazonas state, Brazil, and from Novo Recreio, Guarulhos, Brazil. Last but not least, to those who represent pure love and inspiration: Luciane Viero Mutti, Henrique Mutti Giatti, and Bibiana Mutti Giatti.

Contents

Chapter 1
Introduction: The Relevance of Participatory Approaches Towards Contemporary Dilemmas

This book discusses efforts around science–society interactions in a contemporary world of uncertainties and significant recognition of complexity. The background is based on the current dilemma of socio-environmental and the following public health concerns, but the main issue is to explore how participatory research can be relevant in the search and the need for more social involvement concerning knowledge production, validation, applicability, and diversity. Besides arguing that it is necessary to explore many different layers of determining factors of social and environmental vulnerabilities, the relationship of science with society and the respective domains of nonacademic knowledge and social practices receives primary focus to bring criticism and support to enhance several nuances and possible applications of participatory research.

The principal motivation is to revisit some remarkable and still bright ideas of Paulo Freire, a prominent Brazilian philosopher and educator, in his classic *Pedagogy of the Oppressed* (Freire 2000, 2017). This enthusiastic reference book is proposed for a reinterpretation in the face of transformations and turnarounds imposed by the current science–society interactions and dilemmas. Although this seminal book was firstly published 50 years ago, the vitality of its premises can be certified by its still growing citations and the continuation of profound social and health iniquities characterized by lack of empowerment and scenarios of oppression and marginalization.

Actually, *Pedagogy of the Oppressed* came before the Chernobyl disaster and the respective criticism of the World Risk Society (Beck 2008). It also came before the ethical and scientific uncertainties of developing and producing genetically modified organisms and sadly and surprisingly before the discovery of *prion*, a rising threat and a collateral effect of modernization and application of excessively confident technical and scientific assumptions (De Marchi and Ravetz 1999). Indeed, *Pedagogy of the Oppressed* was also produced and published in a historical moment in which unshakable trust predominantly guided the relationship between science and society. Moreover, such tendency reproduces the hegemonic establishment of academic knowledge in substantial intercourse with certainty and confidence, which

L. L. Giatti, *Participatory Research in the Post-Normal Age*,
https://doi.org/10.1007/978-3-030-27924-0_1

can also be considered as an instrument of power concentration even since its development and acceptance of specific paradigms (Foucault 1980; de Sousa Santos 2009a; Hall 2015; Leff 2017).

In the 1970s, science used to be, as the positivist tradition, a continuous process of specialization within the academic peer communities model of paradigm reproduction as described by Thomas Kuhn (1992), strengthening the perspectives of certainties throughout a problem-solving process. In the field of public health, for example, it is predominantly believed that communicable diseases would be eradicated, something that has never happened until now. Nowadays, we can envisage the current recognition of multifactorial and ecological dynamics involving causative agents, susceptible populations, global and climate changes, migrations, urbanization, behavioral changes, environmental impacts, emergent properties, mutations, and other intrinsic factors undermining unpredictable contexts (Patz et al. 2004; Smith and Ezzati 2005; McMichael et al. 2006; Charron 2012).

Indeed, since the late twentieth century, we have experienced a historical process in which strong criticism has emerged from questioning scientific certainties, somehow strongly motivated by collateral effects of modernity and related respective scientific enterprises. In this scenario, the issue of complexity became to be understood as a challenge to integrate that positivist fragmented scientific knowledge. This added to the rise of respective new epistemological contributions, recognition and acceptance of ambivalence (Bauman 1999), need for interdisciplinary and other related approaches (Morin 2010), reconnaissance and management of uncertainties (Ravetz 2004), and the understanding that some revolutionary scientific innovation can bring new and systemic risks, sometimes associated with unknown and emergent sort of consequences, for those with previous nonexistent preparedness (Beck 2008). Also, the dimensions and scales of the contemporary crisis surpass previous ecological understandings, so as the realization of the great acceleration with the extent of damages never seen before (Steffen et al. 2015), crossing of planetary boundaries (Rockström et al. 2009), and exhibiting the interconnections of scarcities on human needs and vulnerabilities (Hoff 2011). These worrying pieces integrate themselves as we realize the amplitude and unprecedented constraints on the denomination of the Anthropocene (Crutzen 2002).

The contemporary intertwined problems, in the face of the traditional relationship of academic knowledge, decision-making, and societal needs, have also pushed processes of legitimate social control of quality (Gibbons et al. 1994). This has also demonstrated new forms of production and appropriation of knowledge, followed by characterizing ways of validation that are correspondent to social needs, concerns, and accreditation. This new mode of knowledge production and validation has been conceived to be socially robust and targeted to applicability (Gibbons 1999).

Of course, it is not merely an idea that society is questioning the quality of scientific endeavor or methodological assurance and developments. Actually, this a process in which people are appropriating of science and then searching for better protagonism in decisions and choices made on scientific support, as well as reflecting about the applicability of science outcomes and statements. However, such democratic developments are not generally the rule. So, there are many more challenges in this scope of dealing with current dilemma and promoting more knowledge democracy (de Sousa Santos 2009a; Hall 2015).

It is relevant to mention two fundamental movements that are acquiring representativity in recognition of complexity and certainty crisis. The first is related to an internal academic response to the traditional hyperspecialized and fragmented way of producing knowledge in the face of new and emergent problems. The second is represented by the imperative process of cognitive inclusion (de Sousa Santos 2007; de Sousa Santos 2009b), as claim for social justice through democratizing protagonism in the science–society relationship about contemporary crisis and challenges.

Concerning the internal academic responses to complexity, the recognized multicausality of complex issues clearly demands the integration of different kinds of scientific knowledge, and then multi- or interdisciplinary approaches were needed to cope with problems like the emergence of an infectious disease caused by ecological disturbances associated with economic development and populational behavioral changes. In this hypothetical example, a perspective of knowledge integration through sharing methodological strategies and then bringing possibilities of more systemic understanding has been recognized, as typical when applying interdisciplinarity, which can be conceived to be a manner to reconnect knowledge that was separated into the scientific subjects (de Alvarenga et al. 2015). In my opinion, this kind of response to the current scientific dilemma is a legitimate demand as well as a self-criticism of academics to repair the losses caused by the fragmentation of knowledge, besides the outstanding achievements of this process.

Indeed, the process of hyperspecialization of science allowed inestimable advances on one hand, but on the other, it constituted weakness to deal with those intertwined and multifactorial issues. Somehow, although not hegemonic, interdisciplinary research appears as a viable and growing alternative (Van Noorden 2015). One segment of my particular interest concerning the interdisciplinary framework is that one dedicated to conceive, study, and interact with social-ecological systems—SES—mainly concerning the challenging role of multiple understandings on dynamics and interactions like those related to resilience, adaptability, traditional knowledge, feedback learning, and transformability (Berkes et al. 2000; Folke et al. 2010).

SES approach seems to be challenging on one hand for its nature of being originated from ecological studies but then applied to socio-environmental increasing emergent complexities, inherently demanding methodological and conceptual integration. In that direction, there is a daunting concern to avoid simplification regarding ecological concepts or interpretations. That is relevant for not reducing the condition of subjectivity and heterogeneity within those social units to be studied. For example, an important concept to be explored within SES approach is resilience, but it is known that some conceptualization of resilience devoted to cities, for instance, can obfuscate deep social inequalities (Meerow and Newell 2016), as well as the consequences in health- and environment-related risks (Smith and Ezzati 2005).

Besides resilience, another essential concept derived from SES approach to be addressed is diversity. So it is fascinating to push a contemporary reflection about what can be the role of diversity in a SES, mainly in consideration of a property of constant human capacity of creating alternatives that corroborate to a process of acceleration of adaptability (Folke et al. 2010; Moran 2018). In this sense, there is a fundamental concern based in the ability to create alternatives, even in highly vulnerable circumstances, establishing social practices associated with respective knowings. The dynamic and creative process of producing doings and knowings can bring innovation for dealing with apparently chaotic situations, and then it sheds light on the importance and applicability of common sense and popular knowledge (Magnani 2002; de Sousa Santos 2007; Schatzki 2015).

Recognizing the key importance of those knowings and doings, representing common sense, popular knowledge or nonacademic knowledge, allows us to consider that for overlapped problems coming from global crises to local unfoldings—as global environmental changes bring higher risks for communities in association with multilayered vulnerabilities, such as disasters and epidemics—it engenders a variety of responses conditioned to the community's particular features, material possibilities, previous cultural backgrounds, possibility of partnerships and cooperations, public policies opportunities, among other local strengths or weaknesses.

Therefore, the valuation of nonacademic knowledge rises here as a need to deal with the complexity of multilevel problems. However, by contrast, it is also a matter of cognitive justice and empowerment for those who have been marginalized for not dominating the hegemonic scientific knowledge. Boaventura de Sousa Santos has brought a valuable contribution in this sense, calling attention to the idea that to bring social justice it is also necessary to promote cognitive justice. This assumption comes from the realization that the consecration of scientific as the dominant knowledge guided a colonizing process by making all the other forms of knowledge peripheral. Then, there is a need, on one side to recognize the importance and applicability of other kinds of knowledge, and on the other side to foster cognitive justice. Indeed, that corresponds to the desired conjuncture of knowledge democracy (de Sousa Santos 2007, 2009b).

Coming back to the current process of changes considering the relationship between science and society in the face of environmental and health crises, there is a very fundamental criticism to introduce. That is the concept of post-normal science, which a rises from questioning the traditional relation of science and decision-making, then highlighting the uncertainties in opposition of the traditional assumptions of certainty of knowledge to control the natural world. The so-called post-normal problems are complex and characterized by uncertain facts, values in dispute, high stakes, and the need for urgent decisions. The perspective and critic established by post-normal science emphasizes that in front of uncertainties it is observed that scientific communities cannot recognize certain lack of competence, resulting in ignorance, postulates contaminated with value judgment, and, therefore, undermining of confidence. Besides, it is also related to decisions not entirely aware of the possibility of collateral effects and systemic unknown risks (Funtowicz and Ravetz 1993, 2003).

In effect, post-normal science was first mentioned by Silvio Funtowicz and Jerome Ravetz in 1990; since then many developments occurred in the sense of its interpretation, but it did not bring the foundation of a new methodological approach or a new form to produce science. Instead, the theory of post-normal science evolved focusing on the social reality of controversy and dispute around uncertainties and interests, somehow mediating conflicts and erosion of trust between academics and the rest of the society. Thus, post-normal science does not bring recipes for success, and so, contributes to understanding why some stated recipes often come into inadequate in front of multilayered and complex problems, requiring changes in institutions and individual and group mentality, what should be targeted by new scientific educational stances, awareness of uncertainties, and science limitations (Strand 2017).

Maybe the most relevant aspect to be considered here is the presupposition of a more democratic process of quality control related to decisions made on scientific statements about complex problems. In the traditional mainstream production of knowledge, quality assessment is a matter of critical scrutiny by researchers themselves (Funtowicz and Ravetz 2003), and this is characteristic of the "normal science," as being related to scientific training under a specific consolidated paradigm, reproduced inside scientific communities under respective rules and authority (Kuhn 1992). In this sense, considering the limits of uncertainties and the need to bring stakeholders, those implied in the decisions or possible consequences must participate in the decision processes through what has been called the extended peer community (Funtowicz and Ravetz 1993). This proposition is entirely democratic, but besides, it is also a very sensitive assertiveness. Once there is not enough knowledge or recognition about possible collateral effects, systemic risks and emergent properties, like new technologies, must be analyzed through inclusive processes of decision-making, with consciousness about the level of stakes, disputes, ambivalence, and scientific limitations (Ravetz 2004).

Indeed, the extended peer community can also be related to sustainability by two different dimensions, which can be on regard of precaution to avoid ecological imbalances and health-related risks, as well as concerning social stability, in consideration that emergent crisis entailed by approaches of "applied science" to post-normal problems can result in severe consequences for or ruptures in governance structures. Thus, in the post-normal science proposal, there is an imperative for extending the peer community beyond the conventional research peers and industrial sponsors, because conventionally the deliverables of normal science have been deployed in the policy process, and then a broad range of social actors must become appropriately involved in consequent unfolding (De Marchi and Ravetz 1999; Funtowicz and Ravetz 2003).

However, extending peer communities and promoting knowledge democracy converges with sharing power and making permeable the ostensibly policed frontiers that traditionally segregate and marginalize all sort of knowledge distinguished from scientific (de Sousa Santos 2009a; Hall 2015). In the scientific historical development, there is always indication of correspondence between relations of power and relations of meanings, and the consecration of any scientific truth can be understood in the relation of whom such truth serves (Foucault 1980). Nowadays, with the crisis of certainties, and the new magnitude and dimensions of phenomena, a different relation of oppression can be acknowledged. It is evident when just some influential people or institutions can appropriate science in order to apply "normal" judgments favoring their own stakes, in detriment of the whole society that can be obligated to carry on possible systemic consequences obfuscated by ignorance and uncertainty.

Coming back to Frerian concepts (Freire 2000), in the struggle for liberation from oppressive structures, people must reconstruct themselves in an ongoing reflection employing self-recognition within the world in which they live. In this case, a world currently influenced by post-normal dilemmas, where there are uncertainties, high values and stakes in dispute, and also the need for urgent decisions to cope with unknown unfoldings of modern emergent risks (Funtowicz and Ravetz 1993).

In this sense, I strongly consider that participatory research approaches represent a pathway to deal with these new and urgent demands for better, fairer, and more sustainable relationships among science and society. This is not an argument to depreciate the traditional and specialized production of science; in fact, this is a proposal for better application of science to the global societies' real and contemporary needs.

Moreover, the propositions and criticism applied to this current demand for more collaborative science and society relationship is not only a concern dedicated to the emergent problems of modernity, as genetically modified organisms (GMOs), nuclear technologies, or nanotechnologies. This is also a matter to recognize other levels of complexity within some problems that used to be considered as pure. For example, as it is going to be further addressed, an issue of precarious sanitary conditions in an indigenous land in the Brazilian Amazon appears not only as a lack of infrastructure but also as a problem with entangled causes from cultural, social, economic, and political dimensions. Therefore, participatory research approaches can also help in addressing holistic understandings as well as providing possibilities of empowerment, policy mobilization, ways for cooperation, and partnerships. In this kind of situation, participatory research approaches can bound other knowledges in cooperation with scientific, making possible a necessary collaborative knowledge and involvement, as well as promoting cognitive justice and ecology of knowledge (de Sousa Santos 2009a; de Toledo and Giatti 2014; Giatti et al. 2014).

Participatory approaches will be addressed in a broader sense in this book, but mainly in order to stress the importance and the ongoing challenge to promote research approaches that can recognize and favor interactions among academics and lay people, bringing opportunities to aggregate nonacademic knowledge in the process of creating new hybrid and collaborative knowledge. Also, there is a premise to explore the role of participatory approaches for empowering and pushing social engagement in the face of complex contemporary questions and decisions on uncertain issues. Moreover, there is concern about cognitive inclusion related to the perspective of social justice as well as its relevance regarding the diversity of social practices and knowledge as to pave pathways for sustainability.

Because of the subject of discussion, which is the socio-environmental and health-related problems, I focus on the trajectory of social participation in research with the fundamental principles of the Ottawa Charter Health Promotion call for community engagement (Ottawa Charter 1986), but always having in mind the previous emancipatory philosophy of Paulo Freire. Then, two approaches close to these historical developments are chosen, "Community-Based Participatory Research," with significant experiences from the United States, and "Research-action" in Brazil (from the Portuguese term *pesquisa-ação*). Indeed, there is a broad terminology correlated as "action research," "collaborative research," or "participatory action research," as well as there is a tradition originated in the North with the seminal ideas of Kurt Lewin, and a Frerian tradition more convergent with initiatives taken in the Global South (Wallerstein et al. 2017).

Besides the abundance of labeling and roots, I prefer to keep the focus on the premises of participation of stakeholders and the search for knowledge democracy, especially when coupled with multilayered problems, uncertainties, and stakes in dispute, which refers to post-normal problems. In this sense, that is also possible to discuss approaches or methods that are considered by authors as transdisciplinary (Gibbons et al. 1994; Nowotny 2004); or science-for-policy alternatives (Van den Hove 2007); or as a sort of bottom-up, people-centered alternatives, promoting changes to a reflexive development in social and political sense, anchored in people's subjectivity rather than in structures and institutions distinguished by hegemonic top-down stances (Pieterse 1998).

References

Bauman, Z. (1999). *Modernidade e ambivalência*. Rio de Janeiro: Zahar.

Beck, U. (2008). *La Sociedade del Riesgo Mundial: em busca de la seguridade*. Barcelona: Paidós.

Berkes, F., Colding, J., & Folke, C. (2000). Rediscovery of traditional ecological knowledge as adaptive management. *Ecological Applications, 10*, 1251–1262.

Charron, D. F. (2012). Ecosystem approaches to health for a global sustainability agenda. *EcoHealth, 9*, 256–266.

Crutzen, P. J. (2002). Geology of mankind. *Nature, 415*, 23.

de Alvarenga, A. T., de Souza Alvarez, A., Sommerman, A., & Philippi, A., Jr. (2015). Capítulo 2 Interdisciplinaridade e transdisciplinaridade nas tramas da complexidade e desafios aos processos investigativos. In A. Philippi Jr. & V. Fernandes (Eds.), *Práticas da interdisciplinaridade no ensino e pesquisa* (pp. 37–89). Barueri: Manole.

De Marchi, B., & Ravetz, J. R. (1999). Risk management and governance: A post-normal science approach. *Futures, 31*, 743–757.

de Sousa Santos, B. (2007). Para além do pensamento abissal: das linhas globais a uma ecologia de saberes. *Revista Crítica de Ciências Sociais, 78*, 3–46.

de Sousa Santos, B. (2009a). *Una epistemología del sur: la reinvención del conocimiento y la emancipación social*. Mérida: Siglo XXI.

de Sousa Santos, B. (2009b). *Um discurso sobre as ciências* (6th ed.). São Paulo: Cortez.

de Toledo, R. F., & Giatti, L. L. (2014). Challenges to participation in action research. *Health Promotion International, 30*, 162–173.

Folke, C., Carpenter, S. R., Walker, B., et al. (2010). Resilience thinking: Integrating resilience, adaptability and transformability. *Ecology and Society, 15*, 20.
Foucault, M. (1980). *Power/knowledge. Selected Interviews and Other Writings of Michel Foucault*. New York: Pantheon Books.
Freire, P. (2000). Pedagogy of the oppressed (M. B. Ramos, Trans.; D. Macedo, introduction). 30th anniversary ed. London: The Continuum International Publishing Group Inc.
Freire, P. (2017). *Pedagogy of the oppressed* (64th ed.). Brasil: Paz e Terra.
Funtowicz, S. O., & Ravetz, J. R. (1993). Science for the post-normal age. *Futures, 25*, 739–755.
Funtowicz, S., & Ravetz, J. (2003). Post-normal science. In: International Society for Ecological Economics (Ed.). Online Encyclopedia of Ecological Economics at http://www.ecoeco.org/publica/encyc.htm
Giatti, L. L., Landin, R., & de Toledo, R. F. (2014). Aplicabilidade da ecologia de saberes em saúde e ambiente e sua permeabilidade na produção acadêmica. *Ciência & Saúde Coletiva, 19*, 4091–4102.
Gibbons, M. (1999). Science's new social contract with society. *Nature, 402*, C81.
Gibbons, M., Limoges, C., Nowotny, H., et al. (1994). *The new production of knowledge: The dynamics of science and research in contemporary societies*. Thousand Oaks: Sage.
Hall, B. (2015). Beyond epistemicide: Knowledge democracy and higher education.
Hoff, H. (2011). Understanding the nexus: Background paper for the Bonn2011 Nexus Conference. SEI.
Kuhn, T. A. (1992). *A estrutura das revoluções científicas*. São Paulo: Perspectiva.
Leff, E. (2017). Power-knowledge relations in the field of political ecology. *Ambiente & Sociedade, 20*, 225–256.
Magnani, J. G. C. (2002). De perto e de dentro: notas para uma etnografia urbana. *RBCS, 17*, 11–29.
McMichael, A. J., Woodruff, R. E., & Hales, S. (2006). Climate change and human health: Present and future risks. *The Lancet, 367*, 859–869.
Meerow, S., & Newell, J. P. (2016). Urban resilience for whom, what, when, where, and why? *Urban Geography*, 1–21.
Moran, E. (2018). *Human adaptability, student economy edition: An introduction to ecological anthropology*. New York: Routledge.
Morin, E. (2010). *Ciência com consciência* (14th ed.). Rio de Janeiro: Bertrand Brasil.
Nowotny, H. (2004). The potential of transdisciplinarity. In H. Dunin-Woyseth & M. Nielsen (Eds.), *Transdisciplinarity: Making professions and the new mode of knowledge production, the Nordic reader* (pp. 10–19). Oslo: Oslo School of Architecture.
Ottawa Charter. (1986). Ottawa Charter for Health Promotion. First International Conference on Health Promotion, 17–21 November 1986, Ottawa, Canada. Retrieved June 26, 2019, from https://www.who.int/healthpromotion/conferences/previous/ottawa/en/
Patz, J. A., Daszak, P., Tabor, G. M., et al. (2004). Unhealthy landscapes: Policy recommendations on land use change and infectious disease emergence. *Environmental Health Perspectives, 112*, 1092–1098.
Pieterse, J. N. (1998). My paradigm or yours? Alternative development, post-development, reflexive development. *Development and Change, 29*, 343–373.
Ravetz, J. (2004). The post-normal science of precaution. *Futures, 36*, 347–357.
Rockström, J., Steffen, W., Noone, K., et al. (2009). A safe operating space for humanity. *Nature, 461*, 472.
Schatzki, T. (2015). *Spaces of practices and of large social phenomena*. Montreal: Espaces Temps.
Smith, K. R., & Ezzati, M. (2005). How environmental health risks change with development: The epidemiologic and environmental risk transitions revisited. *Annual Review of Environment and Resources, 30*, 291–333.
Steffen, W., Broadgate, W., Deutsch, L., et al. (2015). The trajectory of the Anthropocene: The great acceleration. *The Anthropocene Review, 2*, 81–98.
Strand, R. (2017). Post-normal science. In *Routledge Handbook of Ecological Economics* (pp. 288–298). Abingdon: Routledge.

Van den Hove, S. (2007). A rationale for science–policy interfaces. *Futures, 39*, 807–826.
Van Noorden, R. (2015). Interdisciplinary research by the numbers. *Nature News, 525*, 306.
Wallerstein, N., Giatti, L. L., Bógus, C. M., et al. (2017). Shared participatory research principles and methodologies: Perspectives from the USA and Brazil—45 years after Paulo Freire's "pedagogy of the oppressed". *Societies, 7*, 6.

Chapter 2
Insights from the Contemporary Contradictions in Science–Society Relationship

2.1 Damages, Interests, Science Misuse, and Oppression

Besides the importance of scientific advances for providing a better quality of life, innovation, and a massive amount of benefits for humankind, there are possibilities of science to be appropriated through hegemonic and unfair methods, sometimes wicked, engendering deep inequities, domination, and grave lack of accountability. That is characteristic in some antidialogical and oppressive circumstances when scientific knowledge is supposed to be a property of elites or institutions, to be many times applied in opposition to societies' interests, as causing damages for common resources as the environmental ones.

Freire (2000) described the dialogical method as to contribute to a liberation process from oppressive backgrounds, then he conceived a mutually educational practice for bringing effects in the society, recognized the value of different ways to read the world, and enhanced the character of a collaborative knowing. Thus, a dialogical approach is understood to be more symmetric concerning the relationship among social actors involved. In the Freirian approach, there is a premise of teaching and learning simultaneously, for both teachers and students. This makes valuable the previous understandings of the students or the subjects, in the case of participatory research. Indeed, once teaching and learning are preconditioning each other, researching is also conceived as part of the dialogical process of teaching and learning, involving social actors in the process.

Therefore, it is essential to reconsider the conventional hegemonic process of elevating the traditional scientific knowledge in parallel to diminishing and marginalizing other kinds of knowledge (de Sousa Santos 2009a). In fact, the appropriation of scientific knowledge with its powerful rationality, not permeable for other conceptions and ambivalences, also provided grounds for very severe atrocities as the twentieth century's history sadly demonstrates (Bauman 1999).

The extent of asymmetries is so acute that even when there is an apparent effort to carry out collaborative interactions, for example, involving academics and

L. L. Giatti, *Participatory Research in the Post-Normal Age*,
https://doi.org/10.1007/978-3-030-27924-0_2

ordinary people from a specific vulnerable community, there is a need to understand and deal with a tendentious context of distrust in such interplay. In fact, this kind of incompatibility can disclose different interests among scientists and the community, regularly denoting clear imbalance of power on behalf of the academics (Christopher et al. 2008; Lucero et al. 2017; Wallerstein and Duran 2017).

Dialogical approaches about the contemporary socio-environmental and health dilemma are to contribute for liberation and knowledge democracy, providing means for self-defense on behalf of society. Remarkably, this self-defense is not intended to protect society from science, indeed it is a matter of protecting society from inappropriate use of science due to hidden interests, ignorance, and asymmetrical relations of power and oppression.

To promote a reflection around possibilities, limitations, and applicability for participatory research approaches in this sense, let's start with a very severe and conflicting environmental degradation case settled in Ecuador since the beginning of oil exploitation in that country. In 1967, there was a discovery of a wealthy field of oil beneath the Amazon rainforest in the Easter Ecuadorian territory, which unleashed an oil boom headed by foreign companies with a subsequent contribution of Ecuador's national oil company. Since then, more than two billion barrels of crude oil was extracted but causing the environmental damage spill of millions of gallons of untreated toxic wastes, gas, and oil. All this ecological degradation occurred during decades without control or criminal liability (San Sebastián and Hurtig 2005).

A documentary movie named *Crude* produced by Joe Beringer in 2009 gives a good illustration of the consequences of such a disaster as well as it explores the social struggle of people at risk in asymmetrical correlation with a company's possibilities to argue and to defend itself from juridical accusations. The narrative exposes indigenous and peasant people suffering for decades from harsh health consequences due to pollution, since the beginning of the oil boom. The documentary depicts how difficult it is for local people to attain environmental justice, once there is a need to assign liability on companies, to proceed with environmental remediation, and to deliver health assistance. Otherwise, it remains a condition of insufficiency for accusations substantial enough to occur because of lack of evidence and explanatory causalities.

The company in focus of struggle is Chevron before being named Texaco at the time of the environmental liabilities. One of the worsening values in dispute is around shreds of evidence to blame this international oil company. Chevron started the extensive exploitation and more than 20 years of operation after transferred the competencies to the Ecuadorian oil company. Within this scenario, there are two relevant aspects to difficult causality and liability. First, from a scientific viewpoint, it is not easy to prove whether or what part of the vast amounts of pollution in the environment was deployed by Chevron. Second, it is very clear that at the beginning of 1970s under the national rally for exploiting such a considerable possibility to generate money, no legal agreements or legislation were developed to prevent consequences for the environment or for the indigenous and peasant communities, consisting of those being historically neglected even by government as well by the oil companies.

In the face of the circumstances exposed by the documentary movie, it is possible to verify the company's strategies to escape from accusations and liabilities. In this sense, a testimony of Chevron's scientist chief marks position blaming peasants for consuming water from the rivers that are supposed to be contaminated by fecal coliforms, then making the company to exempting, as well as ignoring the problem of pollution and the respective health effects on exposed people.

There are two worrying questions in this positioning: First, the possibility of the company to appropriate and to produce science oriented to its interests or to give basis to its defensive discourse, making the escape of the liability to sustain itself upon some "scientific statements." Second, the intent of displacing the causality of the problem to other phenomena in which the company's previous attitudes will not be at stake. In fact, there is a remarkable issue in consideration of how to delimit reliable relationships of causes and effects concerning environmental degradation, human expositions, and the occurrence of chronic diseases. Sophisticated epidemiological studies can be required to demonstrate such causality, but, as the indigenous and peasant population of Amazonian Ecuador are poor and marginalized, this environmental and public health concern tend to be neglected. Indeed, those Amazonian people are also excluded by their ways of understanding the context. What becomes terrifying in this dispute is the fact that peasants and their allies have no voice and cognitive space to argue on socio-environmental justice and health equity, since they do not keep causal proofs of ecological degradation and health effects on hegemonic knowledge basis.

After decades of oil exploitation, many attempts of lawsuits and struggle for environmental justice on behalf of local communities, some Ecuadorian NGO's found an opportunity for an epidemiological study in cooperation with the London School of Hygiene and Tropical Medicine (LSHTM) in the early 2000s. The challenge was not only to conduct scientific studies to bring significative results, but also there was an imperative need to involve indigenous and peasant communities in the process to empower them with the scientific outcomes. Popular epidemiology was chosen as an approach that begins in association with the people at risk, changing them from objects to subjects, in a commitment to share power in the research project bringing laypersons' concerns since the preliminary research planning, also reinforcing communitarian engagement as possessing scientific evidence, analyzing data, and appropriating of the produced knowledge.

This participatory enterprise was successful, providing confident results about the consequences of oil pollutants in the environment and health-related impacts. Some results demonstrated that health-adverse effects were toxicological implications, increased risk of spontaneous abortions, and high occurrence of self-reported symptoms associated with exposure, like skin mycosis, tiredness, sore throat, headache, red eyes, and ear pain. Also, there was a comparison of cancer incidences in oil-producing with non-oil-producing areas considering populations of the Amazon region. The amount of data was compiled into a report targeting a general communication within thousands of people living in those risky areas. There was public dissemination of the results as well as academic publications and media diffusion. As a more expressive unfolding, some NGO engaged with the studies together with the Ecuadorian Ministry of Energy and collaborated producing a document named "Environment Regulation for Oil Operations in Ecuador," characterized as an introduction to basic oil exploitation standards and a reference document to drive public policies (San Sebastián and Hurtig 2005).

It is worthy to note such developments as a liberation process against the unfair dispossession of the territory and natural resources associated with aggression and negligence, social exclusion, and misuse of scientific power on the side of oil industry. On the side of indigenous and peasant people, socio-environmental injustices were notably associated with cognitive exclusion, since their ways of reading the world, and their doings and knowings were not eligible to reach the stances of discussion and decision-making. Of course, they were marginalized in the whole process of discovering and exploiting oil, but indeed this process of exclusion was supported by the way they were isolated for not reaching the hegemonic discourse and knowledge. Popular epidemiology, in this case, played a crucial role, validating the local concerns and values by true participation, and it began since the research hypothesis formulation (Brown 1992; Israel et al. 2008). This participatory trial also played a role as converting the rigid frontier of scientific knowledge as more permeable for popular concerns and legitimate interests. Also, this can be seen as a democratization of knowledge in a mode of production that is emerging and allowing broad distribution and appropriation, concentrated in a relatively few institutions (Gibbons et al. 1994).

However, there is an essential thing to remark with regard to the new epidemiologic knowledge produced and the target of its dissemination. As San Sebastián & Hurtig stress: "*This is a point when the popular epidemiology process clashes with the conventional way of disseminating research results where the epidemiologist usually is in charge of when and where the results should be presented. There is a potential tension between the slow dissemination time schedule driven by the organizations of academic institutions and journals and the quick communication requested by activist groups*" (San Sebastián and Hurtig 2005, p. 803). Maybe it is also a matter of the different cognitive and communicative processes and the urgent demand for advocacy. To reach the necessary protagonism, local activists and NGOs had to learn epidemiology, and in this experience, even having an overall contribution by merging their concerns and thoughts with the research dynamics, the product itself is probably much more identified with hegemonic knowledge than with common sense. Of course, this is a meaningful story of empowerment, but even so, we can realize the still happening gap.

Leff (2017) argues that the crisis of ecological policy associated with dispossession and scarcities of natural resources and profound injustices are crisis of civilization rooted in modernity's hegemonic modes of understanding the world coupled with the supremacy of techno-economic rationality. The alternatives for this mainstream structure of power and knowledge can be conceived by the understanding of the social processes within the ecological transformations. In that way, thinking of the world must fundamentally be political and contextualized in theoretical, geographical, and cultural diversities.

The relation among power and knowledge in the sense of environmental and health injustices and the socioecological contemporary dilemma is not only about pursuing or not the keys of hegemonic scientific knowledge. As science is an ongoing process of evolution and permanent revolutions occur through replacement of paradigms (Kuhn 1992), sometimes different paradigms can be related to antagonistic interests, and then the relation among power and knowledge is supposed to be about choosing and advocating for a specific explanatory model (Foucault 1980).

Let's consider two imminent scientific dilemmas with a high degree of uncertainties and stakes, with worrying possibilities of emergent consequences on socioecological systems. One is the issue of climate change in the supposition of anthropogenic causation, with convincing scientific evidence that global warming with the magnitude of a myriad of systemic implications for the biosphere and humankind (Pachauri et al. 2015). The other is the advent of the GMO (genetically modified organisms) as food and crops and their widespread use and consumption, even with high controversies actively dividing in: pro-GMOs science based in preventive and conventional studies guided by cause-and-effect proofs, and anti-GMOs, those that argue the insufficiency of traditional laboratory-controlled trials to unveil the systemic, synergetic, or emergent properties of inherent risks (De Marchi and Ravetz 1999; Ravetz 2004).

In the United States, the positioning of Republican politicians of being very reluctant about the climate hypothesis is remarkable but, in contrast, having a good acceptance for GMOs. So it shows that in front of the main consensus for one or other dilemma, they seem to have their positions mediated by other determining factors. It is worthy to note that a prominent Democrat, Al Gore, headed a substantial effort to politicize the climate change debate. Another significative issue in the right or left positioning about such paradigms is that the Republicans are conservative and continuously defensive against any assumptions or governmental actions to interfere in the market, diminishing citizens' liberty of choice (Hoffman 2015).

The acceptance of a specific paradigm can be determined by a great variety of circumstances and interests, but, of course, this is not merely steered by scientific merit. Indeed, considering the intrinsic perspective of uncertainties, both for climate change as for GMO's adoption, the previous analysis allows the recognition that there is possible quality control for confidence interval within both different paradigms. Therefore, the prevailing procedure of quality control and decision-making has not occurred in collaboration with a diverse range of stakeholders, mainly excluding some of those that can be affected by prospective side effects (Ravetz 2004).

A prominent biologist Ernest Mayr (2005) stressed, considering Darwin's theories, that for decades three or four paradigms for the theory of evolution have coexisted, interplaying through criticisms and also brokering possibilities of acceptance, in this case, because of the very delicate situation regarding antagonisms with societies' religious beliefs. Kuhn (1992) also remarked the chance of different paradigms in coexistence, but somehow it also seems to be a matter of conflict among peer communities.

John Snow was a primary author and researcher in the area of public health, his nineteenth-century classic *On the Mode of Communication of Cholera* (Snow 1999) brought creativity in investigation tools and talent to raise a new paradigm of epidemic causality, in this case with evidence of biological agent existence and water propagation. As Johnson describes in his exciting and well-documented thriller *The Ghost Map* (Johnson 2008), by means of the remnant miasma theory of the nineteenth century, Snow's sagacity encountered considerable resistance to being accepted by the scientific community. The great success and dissemination of the miasma theory supported its application in controversial situations. Then it gave the basis for a system of water supply that ignored the contamination of cholera, and it caused a new geographically spread pattern of the disease, also providing a feedback for the burial of this outdated paradigm.

But it is important to note that there can be resistance for paradigms acceptance also among society. Even when there is a governmental adoption of scientific innovations, a variety of circumstances and reasons can confront such public policies based in science directives. A historical public health case took place in Brazil at the beginning of the twentieth century. The "Vaccine revolt" was an extreme social struggle against the introduction of mass immunization against smallpox imposed as obligatory by the government in 1904, when the Rio de Janeiro city was paralyzed with state of siege decreed. Even with the incidence of thousands of smallpox cases registered in that year, population judged the imposition as a very violent invasion of privacy, besides the mistrust on the effectiveness of the vaccination (Hochman 2011).

Maybe this case seems to be a "thing of the past," but history repeats itself. Since 2017, a reemergence of yellow fever has been in a high chance of re-urbanization in the southeastern Brazilian region, even in São Paulo city with more than 11 million inhabitants. Yellow fever is recognized because of its high potential for lethality, and one very relevant measure to prevent the risk of urban transmission is a mass vaccination. Regularly, only people living in risk areas close to natural reservoirs of the disease receive the immunization. Then, there were two combined problems: lack of enough vaccine shots and peoples mistrust on the quality of the vaccines, mainly because of a procedure of fractionation of shots necessary to promote higher population coverage. Another similar case has been measles reemergence. In Europe, a recent trend of growing cases of measles astonishes when from 2016 to 2017 the number of cases increased fourfold. The causes are strongly associated with the reduction of vaccination coverage, sometimes among vulnerable groups like immigrants, interruptions in vaccine supply, or underperforming disease surveillance systems (WHO 2018). A safe coverage for avoiding measles outbreaks is considered to be 95% with two doses of a measles-mumps-rubella vaccine (MMR) in all population groups and all geographical areas. But there has been evidence that one of the reasons for coverage reduction is related to the fact that people of the current generations have not perceived this disease as a threat, this is a juncture favoring an antivaccination attitude sometimes supported by philosophical or even religious beliefs (Carrillo-Santisteve and Lopalco 2012).

Coming back to the recent Brazilian case of yellow fever, the internet through social networks played an adverse role questioning the quality of vaccines, facilitating dissemination of false evidence and misinformation about the unlikely risk of developing the disease, and dying after receiving the immunization. In this sense, Hoffman (2015) emphasizes that internet and social media would be considered as a substantive tool for democratized knowledge. However, instead of making us more informed, the internet just made us more confident in certainty, once it allows us to find those groups and information to support what we want. Internet and social media have been a possibility for "tribalism" of purposes and ideas, not necessarily an opportunity to open our minds.

But the dynamics involving science appropriation are not only about misuse, mistakes, and hidden interests. Sometimes appropriate science-based decisions with high confidence and evident postures for favoring the majority of the population can be refused by society. Of course, to a certain degree, it was the case of "Vaccine revolt" in Brazil's early twentieth century, mentioned above.

Besides, an admirable case is described as a current posture of resistance against scientific advising for policy. Peter Gluckman, in 2009 newly appointed as first science adviser to the Prime Minister of New Zealand, related that although such a recommendation is an issue under his expertise, New Zealand's food industry would not be required to add folate to flour-based products. This measure would be, as already implemented in many countries, directed at reducing risks of neural-tube defects in newborns. Despite the scientific confidence in this sense, with support from applied cases, a surprising justification arose from public opinion for nonacceptance: various groups didn't want to have their food supply turned into medicine (Gluckman 2014b). For Gibbons (1999), the current process of science to be considered as reliable is not merely a matter of communication, as in the traditional and historical relationship with the society based on confidence and incontestable truths. Today, a new mode of interaction engenders two kinds of the validation processes, the first is conventional inside the laboratory and with scientific communities, and the other is outside, with the society. Then, it is supposed to occur involving social actors, which can corroborate with contestation of any scientific application. This new mode of interaction is considered to be a socially robust knowledge production.

Referring to post-normal science, Gluckman (2014a) adds that science advice, as an evidence-based policy component, does not generally deal with easy issues with strait technical solutions. In effect, it deals with sensitive matters that besides inevitable association with uncertainty degrees, also embodies high public concerns as well as considerable scientific and political complexity.

Science evolves through paradigms and choosing and applying some paradigm is not only a question of confidence, but in this sense, there is also an intrinsic dimension of political choice and intrinsic power and interests (Foucault 1980). Thus, the perspective of applying or accepting some paradigm of a scientific-based decision is related to power relations and disputes, but indeed, there can be some situations of very asymmetrical possibilities concerning how to appropriate science, and this can be established through oppressive scenarios. An excellent example is the Ecuadorian oil scandal, in which many years of social mobilization were necessary, but a new perspective arose only when appropriating hegemonic discourse by means of popular epidemiology.

Sometimes, as in New Zealand's folate addiction refusal, the situations are not about misuse of science but the counterpoint of a moral legitimate choice, since people were not putting scientific advice in doubt. They probably decided for the right to have the integrity of their food, also considering that there would be other possibilities for the same prevention against newborn defects. Particularly, this case sounds like an excellent example of knowledge democratization. Nonetheless, I would argue that behind these enrollments, knowledge democracy and social empowerment would be a prerequisite.

In other conditions, there can be the misuse of science or scientific paradigms even by decision-makers or citizens. Such circumstances, as in wrong policy decisions or mainly in social choices, like the antivaccination behavior are relevant to stress that in this book I do not consider that common sense is a right or must be positioned over the scientific thought. The main point is that common sense or other nonacademic knowledge is essential in the complex process of applying science to a necessary context of controversy and values in dispute. For that, it is worthy to consider cognitive inclusion (de Sousa Santos 2007) as to pave ways for more sustainable arrangements, to make better choices on uncertainties, to prevent oppression, and to attain science's new social contract (Gibbons 1999).

Once, conventionally, there is an abyssal frontier between science and common sense (de Sousa Santos 2004; 2009a), a bridge between these two separate worlds can be built through participatory approaches. In a variety of possibilities to promote collaborative knowledge, dialogical interaction, reciprocity, and trust, the application of successive participatory research tools in a feedback process (List 2006; Christopher et al. 2008; de Toledo and Giatti 2014) can play a decisive role in this sense.

Participatory research approaches can contribute to better and inclusive scientific decision-making in the face of uncertainties (Van den Hove 2000); can promote a kind of science literacy among laypersons to deliver empowerment against oppression and oversights (Wallerstein and Duran 2010; Wallerstein et al. 2017); can merge sanitary (scientific) discourses with cosmological indigenous concepts in order to bring new, collaborative, and decisive knowledge (Giatti et al. 2014); can promote health education in relation to complex and under dispute issues (Querol et al. 2011; Macaia et al. 2018); and above all, can make the membrane of hegemonic knowledge permeable and sensitive for the importance of other forms of knowledge, and this can be understood as a notable process of humanization for the academic ivory tower (de Sousa Santos 2009b).

For Wallerstein and Duran (2010), community-based participatory research can be viewed as an emerging transformative research paradigm, because it can cope with fundamental challenges in order to strengthen communities in the processes of reciprocal knowledge translations with academics for collaborative development, interventions, influence in policies, and reduction of health inequities. Some of these challenges are the acceptance and integration of culturally based evidence, as considering relevant some local explanatory models; the alternative of external validity for scientific discourses by means of recognizing and favoring community health priorities and local possibilities to adapt to interventions; and the rupture with the conventional scientific language that means dominance, and it can be achieved by translating findings to local rationalities associated with real-world constraints like culture variability, resources, organizational factors, and research acceptance.

In the same direction, a broad range of participatory research approaches can also be eligible for attending the post-normal science criticism for helping better scientific training (Strand 2017), contributing for other judgments on uncertainties, facilitating broader quality control, and so making feasible the extended peer community. From the academic side, the stance of recognizing scientific limits and the perspective of stakeholders' validation for knowledge production and application can represent an alternative to breaking the traditional anti-dialogical relationship with society. As Paulo Freire (2000) assertively described, the anti-dialogical banking education is a practice in which the discourse, as a gift or imposition, is to be stored by the students, and the analogy to be placed here is that science produces discourses to be as well delivered and accepted by society. Then, a dialogical relationship among science and society should be necessarily a process of societal questioning, collaborative problem-solving, democratization of knowledge production, and a breakthrough of the prescriptive academic tradition.

Indeed, I argue that this comparison is worthwhile as having the academic as the teacher and the society as the student. This is not a matter of correct or incorrect, or up-to-date or obsolete scientific assumptions. This is a question of how society is to appropriate scientific production in a reflexive and symmetrical process, considering limits, expectations, constraints, and demands. On the other hand, as participatory research also aims at transforming the researcher (Brydon-Miller et al. 2003), the opposite is also true: the community can be the teacher and the researcher a student. Teachers must be facilitators of the pedagogic process in Freirian assumption, so when researchers represent the teacher, they must help to foster the process of interaction and to keep the targets of actions to change reality. When subjects are the teachers, they represent the constant recognition and aggregation of the local cultural background and the permanent encompassing of their wishes and decisions from a democratic perspective. That is the sense of a true dialogical interaction, equity, and symmetry of relationships. Whether traditionally science is to store statements on society, then we see a concrete situation of oppression, and the revolution in this sense is just the perspective of a dialogical relationship.

In convergence with the Freirian proposal of libertarian pedagogy, a process ceasing cultural domination happens through a permanent praxis in which those oppressed commit themselves to transformation, in this sense, society provided with common sense knowings must no longer be marginalized. In fact, a continuous process of interaction should enable mutual recognition and learning. Then, science and society from their different points of view must learn continually from teaching mutually. For dialogical scientific teaching, it is imperative to establish a process of learning and knowing that consistently involves theorizing about the experiences shared by academics and society in the ongoing process. But, of course, it is also a matter of sharing power since the standard configuration is through domination and dispossession, with science studying society, not learning collectively and not being ascribed of extended validation on behalf of stakeholders.

2.2 Browsing from Simple to Complex

As mentioned before, the post-normal criticism is very relevant to support the need and the right for knowledge democracy so as to promote the extended peer communities. This kind of broad stakeholders' involvement is argued for Funtowicz and Ravetz (1993) as a demand for fairer, safer, and conscious decision-making in the face of those so-called post-normal problems. However, tellingly, the ascension of such concepts is strongly related to the certainties crisis, mainly in the drawing of the new age of high technologies and the perspective of systemic and unknown possibilities of consequences, like technological catastrophes, epidemics, ecological imbalances, or disasters. In contrast, post-normal science has also played a role in analyzing natural disasters with systemic and enlarged chains of consequences, as well as regarding the unpredictable premise in such (Benessia and De Marchi 2017; Tsukahara 2017).

In this sense, the assumptions of post-normal science have demonstrated the limits of high complexity contexts, then characterizing such post-normal problems as being related to unpredictability, incomplete control, plurality of legitimate perspectives, and conflicting interests. Post-normal problems are also classically associated with uncertain facts and developments, values in dispute, high stakes, and the need for urgent decisions (Funtowicz and Ravetz 1993).

The proposition of the extended peer community is a transcendent alternative and a key element for managing uncertainties, once this process must be more committed to conscious decisions and recognition of limits than to the search for unshakable truths. It can be understood in parallel with transcending old dichotomies like that of knowledge and ignorance, or natural systems and socio-ecological ones. In effect, it is worthy to recognize that the interactions of human and natural systems have emergent properties and a variety of intrinsic knowings and doings that are conditioned by and determinant of ecosystems and or social spaces (Walker et al. 2004; Folke et al. 2010; Schatzki 2015).

However, the property of transcendence allows us to explore other interdependencies and complexities. There are lots of scientific questions that have had decisive and assertive answers. In this scope, the proposition of post-normal science brings the sort of problems that are supposed to have a resolution within normal science, but somewhat there are other dimensions of determinants to explore even in this very assertive issues. Among them, and with a particular interest in this book, are some issues related to health and basic sanitary conditions. For example, it is very acceptable a straightforward relation of causality regarding gastrointestinal diseases due to a general lack of sanitation, as represented by the absence of flushed toilets, inexistent or inappropriate sewage collection and treatment systems, and environmental exposure of humans to fecal contaminants. Many of the principal biological agents of such gastrointestinal or diarrheal diseases are much known, and their respective transmission mechanisms are entirely described.

Nevertheless, such a massive amount of knowledge delivered for excellent scientific production is not enough to avoid or eradicate intestinal parasites among human populations. Before judging this lateness as a particularity of vulnerable people living in poverty and social exclusion, it is worth to remark that this kind of health concern is still to a certain degree a widespread problem also in developed countries. In effect, the relation of water, sanitation, and hygiene sometimes seems to be like forgotten institutions, and such a condition probably suggests a level of negligence for those related issues (Bartram and Cairncross 2010).

In truth, sanitary conditions are not such a simple issue, and a range of causality layers can be verified in addition to the conventional knowledge concerning respective consequences to human health. Then, this supposed unattractive and not challenging scientific question must be faced with local characteristics, like socio-environmental, historical, and cultural to bring insights about the inherent complexity and the need for more interdisciplinary and participatory approaches. To bring these assumptions closer to pragmatism, a case study in an indigenous community in the Brazilian Amazon Region is explored, as being an experience of studying the multifactorial causes regarding sanitation and health as well as an alternative for building collaborative knowledge, empowerment, and valuable insights for health promotion.

This research experience takes us to a background too distant from urban and modern contexts in which the academic staff is. So far, it can teach us so much because of the dramatic differences to be understood. The investigation took place from 2004 to 2009 in a multi-ethnic agglomeration composed of ten small indigenous communities located in Amazonas State just on the border with Colombia. The investigation site is named Iauaretê—an indigenous nomenclature that means waterfall of the jaguar. The population was of approximately 2700 inhabitants, and the sanitary conditions were expressed by lack of safe water supply, absence of flush toilets, worrying hygiene practices, and general lack of public policies to address such an acute environmental health context (Giatti et al. 2007; de Toledo et al. 2012).

An oversimplified way to address this vulnerable background would be just the provision of water and sanitation improvements, but on one hand, there were general material constraints because of abandonment due to institutional and budget deficiencies, corroborated by the fact that this same sanitary context was widespread in tens of analogous communities in the same territory. On the other hand, socio-cultural conditions were relevant in the chain of determinants of the vulnerable context and those aspects could not be overlapped just for infrastructure. In this sense, the socio-cultural attributes were the main focus of the study, since research-action was applied with the focus on the lack of sanitary conditions and health concerns.

Research-action denomination is a reference to the Brazilian tradition of the similar term in Portuguese: *pesquisa-ação*. This methodology is very compliant with Freirean assumptions regarding a dialogical process involving continuous learning and cooperation among researchers and subjects of the studied problem. As an underpinned definition, Michel Thiollent states that "research-action" is a method of empirical social research carried in narrow association with a collective action or problem-solving, in which researchers and stakeholders are involved in a cooperative or participative manner (Thiollent 2011).

Many fieldwork campaigns were taken, some with 15 days of work reproducing application of participatory research tools through meetings in each one of the small component communities. Some of these tools were talking maps—a graphic representation of environmental health issues through collaborative drawing and explaining; photovoice (or adapted photo panel)—photos produced by the indigenous and brought to the discussion on basic sanitary and health problems, their causes, and possible alternatives for mitigation; and community newspaper—a joint elaboration of a manually produced newspaper focusing on the basic sanitary and health concerns, which was produced and distributed by the indigenous in any one of the Iauaretê's households.

Alongside the research process, some quantitative and qualitative trials, like interviews, questionnaires, parasitological survey, and microbiological analysis of water supply, were applied to get a broad understanding about the wholeness of causalities implicated in the environmental and health local context, then characterizing a mixed method research. Somehow, the participatory research tools were considered to be the conducting axis of the process, making possible the primary targets of dialogical participation in the sense of its pedagogic power, and contributing to social mobilization and empowerment. The participatory process was considered to be cyclic enabling successive phases of planning, acting, and fact-finding, then bringing a contribution to the seminal proposal of action research (Lewin 1946) into a feedback-adaptive practice (de Toledo and Giatti 2014).

This research experience brought a variety of results, sometimes also showing relative contradictions regarding the sociocultural transitions of the studied population. For example, to explain the causes of diarrheal diseases, even having evidence of understandings about the precarious sanitary conditions, the indigenous provided answers like "diarrhea is a spell" or the relatively opposite "we defecate everywhere." The study showed not only contradictions of having or not having appropriation about the sanitary and health mainstream discourse but also depicted how those indegenous people read the world in a transition among their traditional knowledge and the dominant health assumptions. Besides, the dialogical participatory process provided them with opportunities to have reflexive conversations among their communities on issues that had been treated with less importance, making the indigenous to work on joined proposals with the researches as well as building capacity to promote health (Giatti et al. 2007).

The Iauaretê's study also showed disparities within the outcomes accomplished, then pushing preventive alternatives in individual and communitarian level. It also demonstrated the lack of initiatives from the public policies that would be indispensable for implementing basic sanitary infrastructure, that is, water supply and sanitation. In this sense, the indigenous with the support of researchers elaborated a petition to public institutions on their right to have such infrastructure. Therefore, the academic contribution and the scientific background of the study contributed as a support for advocacy in health issues.

In summary of the case study, a research-action process of investigation, as a participatory method dedicated to problem-solving and collaborative knowledge production, is a straightforward possibility to explore different intertwined layers of determinants of problems like sanitation and health concerns. Indeed, in such an approach, it is considered that basic sanitary conditions can be linked to other complexities. Therefore, if research-action is useful to disclose and emphasize complexity, why not consider this kind of approach also to address post-normal problems?

Participatory research approaches are mainly dedicated to addressing inequities in health and environmental-related concerns among minorities, groups in a condition of social exclusion, small communities, rural settlements, or indigenous people. This concern about scale seems to be relevant in the tendency of developing participatory approaches within the contemporary scientific crisis of relationship with society. However, even with a majority of local/small-scale trials, there are some valuable examples of approaches dedicated to larger scales of social issues (like cities, regions, river basins), and sometimes, experiences that deal with wide ranges of stakeholders, embracing the nature of the studied questions, like searching for international or global concerns. That is a relevant point regarding finding approximations about participatory approaches and the particular applicability on those problems raised by post-normal science (Giatti 2013, 2015).

Initiatives of post-normal science applications have occurred traditionally in Europe, and the main guideline for developments in this sense has been the adoption of the precautionary principle to deal with uncertainties and high stakes, but it is clearly related to large-scale and leading-edge matters or highly uncertain issues, like natural disasters and new technologies. In 2014, an international symposium on post-normal science practice was held in the Centre for the Study of the Sciences and the Humanities of the University of Bergen, Norway. The purpose was to bring together practitioners and theorists to critically reflect upon possible implementations and futures work. Then a sort of assumptions arose so as to recognize the need for engaging diverse groups of lay people, academics, and decision-makers to address post-normal problems, reinforcing the proposal of extended peer communities. Moreover, the process of dialoguing with such communities reinforced the idea of considering post-normal science as "*a heuristic device, allowing citizens and decision-makers to consider problems from different perspectives*" (Dankel et al. 2017, p. 2).

In a case of an application that is correspondent to the propositions of post-normal science, Van Den Hove (2000) explored a participatory approach on environmental policy-making that took place between 1997 and 1998 during the last phase of the international negotiations organized by the European Commission related to the Kyoto Conference of the Parties to the UN Framework Convention on Climate Change, and the elaboration of the post-Kyoto commitments. The case study encompassed a rich background concerning the complexity involved, considering uncertainties, perspectives of the irreversibility of damages, and scientific limits to predict the nature and the extent of climate change-related consequences on multiple scales from global to local.

The additional complexity inherent to the social dimension is a relevant issue to be addressed as described, also contributing to justify the need for broad stakeholders' involvement in the debates and decision-making. In this sense, there is a description of a substantive participatory process taken through five workshops with the following social actors: research experts; European Community Climate negotiation team; European Union Member States representatives; other Commission interests; and outside stakeholders including industry, finance, commerce, employment, environment, consumer, and citizen interests. The participation process occurred through workshops as having specific issues to address. Two concerns were raised in this sense, first the importance of different knowledge and expertise to design creative and collaborative alternatives. Second, the necessary recognition that the large amplitude of the climate change-related causes and possible consequences is transcendent to national governments, private actors, and the whole society. Such a cross-cutting characteristic also relates to time scales, like future generations. This complex framework imposes a burden that is impossible to deal with without extensive international and multilevel collaboration, as well as encompassing future scenarios.

The experience also demonstrated that the extensive and intertwined nature of the problem, and the possibility of multiple interpretations of uncertainties, demands a dedicated work on conflict resolution in order to integrate such different value judgments, social representations, and distinct levels and possibilities of risks and vulnerabilities.

In effect, this European experience was very innovative and an excellent contribution. However, it is not necessarily a guideline to manage such vast and complicated amount of factors and social actors' interests and values. More than this, the participatory approach process described gives us some insights on how to build collaborative structures to deal with this prominent contemporary dilemma concerning science and society relationships. Indeed, this studied case underpins the real need to find possibilities for stakeholders' involvement.

Climate change is not only a post-normal problem, it is also one of the broader or maybe the broadest socio-environmental health-related concern that the humankind has ever faced or recognized. According to an impacting and critical text of Hulme (2007), published in the British newspaper "The Guardian," climate change incurs in the danger of a "normal" reading of science, in which prevails the idea that science always can find the truth—or the solution. The nature of this scientific dilemma calls attention to the provisional status of knowledge as well as the perspective that such knowledge can be amended in interaction with society. Indeed, climate change also calls attention to necessary considerations on confidence in science and technology, to possible divergence among the collective action and private enterprise, dependence on funding and quality evaluation. Moreover, climate change enrolments can be related to disputes about scientific truth, possibility of errors, interests, and a myriad of understandings.

Coming back to the possibility of participatory approaches, my personal opinion is that there is much more methodological expertise and criteria in participatory approaches dedicated to the majority of research experiences in local contexts than in the applications that can be understood as to post-normal problems, like involving a broad set of stakeholders to deal with large-scale and leading-edge matters or highly uncertain issues. It can be checked through bibliographic reviews (Giatti 2013, 2015), but, actually, there are two relevant concerns in this sense: On one hand, those appointed post-normal problems are strongly demanding the recognition of the social emergent complexity in terms of dealing with the scientific dilemma, and this makes the imperative of the extended peer communities to build better alternatives. However, maybe there is no substantial provision on how to promote such participatory processes in a satisfactory level of quality to reach sophisticated collaborative arrangements. On the other hand, many contributions and developments in theoretical and methodological frameworks are distinguishable in the participatory approaches like research-action or community-based participatory research, as mentioned before with a majority of experiences among small population groups, or local targeting.

In this sense, the assumption that participatory approaches must be applied to transcend levels of complexity arises again. This kind of interactions must also transcend abyssal ruptures, as to bridge such different kinds of knowledge, like scientific and popular, then contributing for new and collaborative knowledge, mutual learning, and reduction of abyssal disparities. For Boaventura de Sousa Santos, research action, for example, is a powerful instrument to operate throughout the separating border between science and society. Participatory action research can be a mechanism for translating, merging, and promoting relevant interactions among knowledges, it can provide couplings to connect different cognitive domains (de Sousa Santos 2004).

The application of participatory approaches to a problem of low degree of uncertainty like sanitary conditions and health can unveil levels of complexity and causal determinants that could be hidden or overshadowed. Moreover, this kind of local approach, through learning and dialogical interactions, can help to build collaborative solutions to those not so simple contexts. In fact, according to Morin (2010), there are no simple issues, only simplification, and in this sense, the complexity can be understood as interdependencies, which are woven together as fabric. The problem of complexity is not the completeness but the incompleteness of knowledge and the necessary complex thinking that must take into account all the fragments left by the segmented thinking.

Participatory approaches can be a vehicle to browse throughout dimensions of complexity, as so to make possible encompassing incompleteness and apparently hidden determinants. In this perspective of being a vehicle, it is also understood the importance of participatory research to link and make positive interactions among different kinds of knowledge, like academic and popular.

At another extreme, post-normal problems can also benefit from this potential to browse through dimensions of complexity and distinct knowledges. Also, participatory approaches can be applied at the beginning of recognition of a high level of complexity, permeated by uncertainties and stakes. This kind of approach is a mode to promote extended peer communities, but it is relevant to stress that there is a need for finding better developments and spaces for participatory research methods and tools. Maybe the tradition of participation in small communities can teach some relevant lessons to these very concerning issues of the contemporary crisis in the relationship of science with the society.

The more prominent problems and uncertainties are, the higher can be the stakes, and the relative power concentration, as well as the more insuperable is the frontier of science and common sense. If conventionally science policy is not friendly of societal criticism, then in the face of the post-normal problems, there is still a wider significant gap concerning disputes. For that matter, the property of participatory research to build more symmetric dialog within a variety of social actors can also contribute to manage antagonisms and also to provide better accountability. However, the decision and possibility to apply a participatory approach to manage a post-normal issue is a political stance, and it can be related to the stance of sharing power and responsibility.

The proposal of pushing forward participatory approaches for knowledge democracy cannot be confused with refusing science in compliance with the growing pseudoscience or post-truth postures associated with the nowadays conservative right-wing politics. The denialism of science has been very significative on issues of biodiversity, sustainability, vaccination, climate change, and biological evolution, and many times this is entirely related to environmental policies somehow considered as threatening the traditional ways of Western progress (Jacques et al. 2008; Hansson 2017).

The assumptions of post-normal science can be useful also for this analysis, avoiding misunderstandings with science denialism. According to the highest levels of uncertainties and stakes, the post-normal problems are in a sector in which there is an imperative for recognizing the limits of science, and not merely denying the scientific assumptions. In this sector of high stakes and ambivalence on values, the broad participation of a variety of social actors with stakes is something necessary because of the decisions to be taken. Those decisions must be much more related to conscious valuations of risks and own perceptions than related to a scientific certainty, which cannot be attained.

Otherwise, when science and decisions are closer to the post-normal vertex as with the high level of certainty, there must be some possible confrontation with science and with the way that science is applied within conflicts of interest and deepening inequities. Again, it is not a matter of anti-science stance against well-established and assertive scientific developments. In this sector of good scientific control of methods and results on related phenomena, sometimes there are overlapping interests of those who have the domain of science on those who have no means to appropriate the hegemonic knowledge to struggle for their self-defense. As mentioned before, even for some surpassed scientific issues, there must be other determinants in the social domain that bring other layers of complexity, and in this sense, participatory approaches can be relevant to promote cognitive justice reducing inequities and fostering balanced application of science.

2.3 Inter-and Transdisciplinarity, and Ecology of Knowledge

For Edgar Morin (2010), the question "*what is science*?" has no scientific answer (p. 119). The meaning of this paradox is the growing extent of incompleteness in parallel with scientific development. Moreover, the concomitance goes further as the unprecedented progress of knowledge raises in correlation with ignorance; the advances in scientific achievements and discoveries reflect in possibilities of harmful and deadly consequences; and finally, the growing power of science unleashes impotence of scientists in the face of the power and extent of scientific outcomes.

These conjectures distinguish the fragmented nature of the scientific development in modernity, and a relevant mark of such scattering is the strong and historical process of disciplinary enclosures and hyperspecialization of the academic culture. The recognition of these enrollments is unequivocal in the threshold of the certainty crisis and the rise of systemic and urgent problems like those characterized as post-normal. The current dilemma involving science, decision-making, and social relationships cannot be tackled once meeting a structure in which scientific knowledge has been reduced into crumbs.

Interdisciplinary and transdisciplinary approaches have been appointed as possibilities to interplay with the nature of wholeness, complexity, and hybridization of problems and related causes in the real world. To a certain degree, these approaches have the promise to rescind the reductionism and the fragmentation of knowledge. Therefore, the need for inter- and transdisciplinarity can be understood as a response to the ongoing cultural revolution that has been followed by new domains of creation (e.g., nanotechnologies), the discovery of new spaces of knowledge, and the growing anthropization of the material world, then posing theoretical and methodological challenges, practical and also conceptual (Raynaut 2011).

Regarding applicability, the interdisciplinary approach aims at relinking knowledge in order to recover from the fragmentation, then transposing the empty spaces among the disciplinary frontiers. This proposal dates back to the 1960s and has been conceived as an alternative method to be complementary and not necessarily competing with the disciplinary tradition. Interdisciplinarity presupposes the production of knowledge about complex phenomena and operates as theoretical, methodological, and technological exchanges creating new narratives (de Alvarenga et al. 2015). Then, it can be conceived as a uniform explicit formulation through discipline-transcending common framework and methods (Gibbons et al. 1994).

Although positivism made its history of fragmentation and knowledge hyperspecialization, transdisciplinarity was present at the beginning and science would not be science without this genesis. However, the modern knowledge statute operated a process of exclusion of subjects through a concentration phenomenon in which the majority of individuals were destitute of the right to have reflections. That was a separation between subject/object, and the current threshold of new scientific knowledge requires the return of the subject as inserted in his culture, in his society, to aggregate from subjectivity (Morin 2010).

Transdisciplinarity can be such a polysemic concept, but in general, it is possible to consider the basic characteristic of being an alternative that goes beyond the scientific disciplines and the knowledge generated from them, therefore transcending the constituted science domain through other forms of knowledge for all of them to be forged in an articulated system (de Alvarenga et al. 2015). A transdisciplinary approach must result in a common theoretical understanding accompanied by mutual interpretation of disciplinary epistemologies. It is a result of overcoming disciplinary modes of problem-solving with the emergence of a new mode of knowledge production based on broader societal and cognitive pressures. In other words, the rise of transdisciplinary initiatives is a legitimate claim from society to the traditional mode of scientific production (Gibbons et al. 1994).

Some requirements in this sense can be needed for transdisciplinary approaches aiming at sustainability, which according to Lang et al. (2012) must be having focus on societal relevant problems; fostering mutual or collaborative learning processes among social actors from outside academia and researchers from different disciplines; and producing knowledge as solution oriented and with respective quality control from the society, as characterizing to become socially robust (Gibbons 1999). In fact, such requirements and background on post-normal problems and complex contemporary issues related to sustainability can be viewed as very similar with the propositions and practices of participatory research (like research-action and CBPR).

Then, there has been this new mode of knowledge production as a process of society to assume a position within scientific discourses applied to decision-making. This kind of relationship, many times as a form of confrontation, stems from crises in public confidence, as in situations like mobilization motivated by lack of trust on some joined science, technology, and market impositions. Many researchers mistake themselves considering this as a refutation of their work, but it is not merely an issue of questioning the quality of scientific disciplinary production. The confrontation in this sense is a legitimate balance of controversy concerning the applicability of science and technology, and this is a process of establishing a socially robust knowledge. For Nowotny (2004), a characteristic of this new kind of knowledge production is transdisciplinarity, having quality control as a relevant criterion, which is not only related to scientific excellence, but also shaped by societal value addiction.

Again it is relevant to remark the perspective of quality control and the extended peer community as a second validation stance and a requirement to deal with post-normal problems. Also, from this particular view, transdisciplinarity must undoubtedly be a standard approach for post-normal science. But, there is a very remarkable problem in this sense that cannot be ignored or simplified: the unfair and abyssal distance of the hegemonic scientific knowledge from other forms of knowledge. Such historical and even deepening cognitive gap is outlined with violence, exclusion, colonialism, and dispossession of cognitive territories (de Sousa Santos 2009a; Hall 2015). In this book, I assume that this gap can be deepening in the context of high interdependency, complexity, and uncertainties of sustainability and health issues, emblematic emerging themes of our contemporary crises.

The provocative and quite necessary reflection raises on the contestation that maybe it is not so easy to perform transdisciplinary approaches since there is an oppressive relationship among those so distant knowledges, specifically on one side the disciplinary science corpus and on the other side all of the nonacademic knowledge. An indicative of disturbance is that uneventfully the outcomes of transdisciplinary approaches have much more similarities with conventional ways of scientific production and somehow those collaborative and transcendent trials commonly have to be validated within the scientific environment.

Maybe the transdisciplinary approaches as commonly recognized can contribute in allowing laypersons to appropriate science in order to context their vulnerability conditions. On the other hand, such premises can pave alternatives for including social actors and their knowledge and perspectives in the process of making the decisions on what is important to them, as well as to allow the mutual learning process, the quality control on the scientific statements, and the production of hybrid adaptive knowledge. Of course, it is an essential outcome with empowerment and advocacy, for example, to marginalized indigenous people, and an excellent case is the popular epidemiology research held in Ecuador dedicated to oil exploitation and environmental and public health-related iniquities (San Sebastián and Hurtig 2005). However, to which degree can we consider that there was a real process of cognitive justice in such participatory research experience? Did the traditional Ecuadorian indigenous' knowledge have a legitimate space regarding creating new, necessary, and good hybrid knowledge? Alternatively, has this process occurred just as an instrument to make laypersons appropriate traditional science and particular methods to protect themselves from the consequences of environmental hazards?

Perhaps, in consideration of other necessary structures for participation and other dialogical endeavors, we should be more careful to accept what is transdisciplinary or not. Alternatives for translation of "languages" (academic to common sense) have also been argued as a relevant stance to make possible interactions among scientific knowledge with other cultures, moral, and values. However, translation in this sense is not a challenge only to make both social actors (academics and society) to speak the same dominant language, which is the scientific. The question is the challenge to build trust employing a reciprocal knowledge translation, and the legitimate result must be hybridization (de Sousa Santos 2004; Wallerstein and Duran 2010; Giatti et al. 2014).

It is worthy to consider that inter- and transdisciplinarity are necessary processes to overlap the fragmentation of traditional ways of academic and hegemonic knowledge production, which is also a form of concentration of power and, sometimes, an oppressive mechanism. Not being a matter of the quality of scientific disciplinary production itself, it is a concern around the interdependencies, complexities of current dilemmas, plus the issue of cognitive justice in the sense of the feasibility of solutions to post-normal problems.

Anyhow, siloed decision-making is also a tradition stemming from disciplinary thinking, and there still is a serious challenge in conceiving parallel interdisciplinary trials in forms of managing complex problems, which must be delivered through intersectoral approaches. For instance, towards public policies on climate change, it is necessary to merge targets in different sectors like energy, public health, and urban transportation. From epistemology to the real-world action, interdisciplinary projects can be friendly to intersectoriality. Moreover, transdisciplinarity promotes knowledge democracy. This requires true social inclusion to encompass cognitive diversities.

In my opinion, inter- and transdisciplinary endeavors are fair and necessary responses from the academics and decision-makers to the real world, and it can also be considered as something to recover the wasted time on the supremacy of scientific disciplinary developments. In other words, inter- and transdisciplinary approaches can be a self-criticism and alternatives from science to pay back for the emergent consequences, negligence of complexities, and isolation caused by mainstream hyperspecialization.

That is why, besides recognizing the relevance of discussion on transdisciplinarity, I do not prefer to classify participatory research dedicated to sustainability and health issues as transdisciplinary. Maybe participatory research targets transdisciplinarity, but reaching it must be something to consider only in the case of substantial cognitive inclusion, a stance that even evaluation parameters can be fuzzy. Therefore, the aspiration here is to keep focus in the process of participatory approaches dedicated to overlap the matter of fragmentation associated with the cognitive exclusion and asymmetrical relationships, under some transdisciplinarity directives. Moreover, a key aspect in this sense is the need to push forward dialogical interactions among academics and social actors, enabling that knowledges from such different natures to interact, coupling in new and hybrid knowledge throughout reciprocal and symmetrical learning processes. For sure, it is not easy to achieve, and a very relevant point must be preventing to see the matter of power imbalance as something implicit and not considered as a determinant. In fact, this matter of asymmetrical and relatively ignored feature must be taken into account as one of the main challenges for participatory research to contribute with post-normal problems.

On these considerations, the idea of the ecology of knowledge seems to be appropriate, because it is supported by the presumption that scientific knowledge is one more and not the only way of producing knowledge. Accordingly, other nonacademic knowledges must gain importance because of their applicability and possibility of fostering equitable interactions and hybrid outcomes (de Sousa Santos 2009a).

Any person has the ability to start reading the world even before reading the words, that is to say, learning to write. People living in a condition of vulnerability with low literacy can also have their reflections and understandings on complex causalities and possible alternatives to survive. Their cultural backgrounds and life experiences support such reflections and understandings, but the development of practices that ignore the common sense understandings are typical of "banking" education, characterized by the imposition of top-down models of problem-solving and rationality. This kind of practice is supported by the hegemony of scientific knowledge, contributing to an oppressive relationship among science decision-making and society. Then, some liberation alternatives and dialogical interactions must be required (Freire 2000). Besides such Freirean assumptions, it is reasonable to presume that the banking relationships with society operate to suffocate the generative capacity of societies to produce a diversity of problem-solving alternatives and knowings, something that should be considered in the current understanding on resilience of socio-ecological systems (Berkes et al. 2000; Walker et al. 2004).

What I argue here is that, in the contemporary crisis of uncertainties, unsustainability, and health-related consequences, this is not only a matter of oppression concerning cognitive exclusion. It is also a question of searching for sustainability within its multiple dimensions, where nonacademic knowledges and practices can be decisive for new and plural alternatives, as well as to promoting liberation, engagement, and communitarian empowerment. This process of "ecologizing" knowledges can be vital even to avoid disasters and to mitigate respective expanded and systemic unfoldings.

2.4 Disasters of Cognitive Exclusion

Extending the peer communities in order to make a better quality control on decisions or even as a way to make more inclusive and fair decisions on post-normal problems can be recommended to deal with the risks of natural or man-made technological disasters. Indeed, some contributions on more integrative and adaptive alternatives for risk governance have also been proposed to include stakeholders' participation in dealing with the nature of complexity, scientific uncertainty, and socio-political ambiguity. Such participatory processes can be relevant to involve different representatives in fair opportunities to connect themselves in decision-making and policy implementation; empowering all actors through the construction of collaborative discourses encompassing a plurality of options, interests, perceptions, concerns, and values; and generating common understanding and learning (Renn 2008; Klinke and Renn 2012; Nederland and Groupe 2013; Linkov et al. 2018).

However, the opposite of nonparticipation seems to be a constant when we observe the background as well as the unfolding of many remarkable disasters. The point to be explored in this sense is the cognitive exclusion that can be related as a worsening variable in two different ways: firstly, in an ex ante scenario in which the lack of involvement of stakeholders (the broad range of social actors to be related to any possible disaster as decision-makers, aid institutions, laypersons who live in any vulnerable context, among others) can be related with lack or inappropriate preparedness or low resilience and responsiveness; secondly, in an ex post scenario, in which the ongoing and systemic extended consequences can also be worsening because of the same lack of involvement, inducing systemic unfoldings.

Indeed, the matter of involvement argued here must be much more in depth than just a process of communication. The real engagement to face the conventional cognitive exclusion must be built in a dialogical process of interactions, fostering trust, reciprocity, commitment, and social learning through participatory-oriented processes (Wals 2007; Christopher et al. 2008). To be dialogical, even the humbler social actors must be involved in the process, having the opportunity, through a self-reflection on their context, to evaluate the risk and to consider which kind of alternatives can be better to them. That is an engagement to build preventive or precautionary stance in convergence with the appropriation of any contingency plan by the stakeholders. That is a mean of making possible, through accessible communication and collaboration, a collective reflection and a fairer negotiation involving different social actors to act on scarcities and distinct needs of a social system. Thus, this kind of social learning can be conceived as a construction, which makes sense for social transformation (Wildemeersch 2007).

On the other hand, the maintenance and reproduction of cognitive exclusion, which can even be materialized through misinformation and lack of transparency, is something to extend the possibility of damages and serious secondary or systemic risks considering the dynamic of a socio-ecological system. That is what we can realize in exploring some remarkable and dramatic disasters of natural, technological, or combined background.

A very iconographic technological disaster at the beginning of a growing global environmental concern was the Seveso case in Italy, 1976 (De Marchi and Ravetz 1999). Due to an increase in pressure associated with an exothermic reaction, the rupture of a safety valve resulted in the escape of a toxic cloud into the air from the ICMESA chemical company. Although the company's managers immediately recognized the problem, local authorities were just gradually informed about the seriousness of the accident. Among other contaminants, the presence of dioxin, known to be extremely dangerous, was identified. Actually, among other evidence dioxin was also known in the 1970s as being a component of "Agent Orange," with the polemic use during the Vietnam War.

The population was also informed late, since the presence of dioxin warning was issued only 9 days after the accident, when the first symptoms had appeared, registering chloracne on the skin of children and deaths of small animals. Just at that time, the main measures were taken as suppression of the industrial activity and erection of fences around the most contaminated zone, as well as the evacuation of a few hundred residents.

The area of the toxic cloud spread was considered to affect 11 municipalities with a population around 220,000, which started to be monitored through long-term epidemiological programs, mainly dedicated to searching for consequences like abortion, malformation, cancer, and deaths, besides the immediate acute consequences. However, even more than 20 years after the accident, the Seveso case is still considered a "modest consequence with lack of "rigorous causal proofs of death and disease," allowing some to state it was "the disaster that never happened" (De Marchi and Ravetz 1999, p. 746).

However, it is worthy to note that things are not merely so simple when involving other kinds of social reactions and developments as in a disaster permeated by fear and doubt. First of all, it is astonishing to realize how far the communication and measures came after the escape of the toxic cloud. After the late society's awareness about the damages, a climate of mistrust took place against the company and the public authorities. The characteristics of the unpredictable level of exposition and the possibility of consequences strengthened the atmosphere of fear and doubt, and then, a series of implications came associated with psychological, social, and economic impacts. Dioxin features made the worsening pressure since it is something with the probability of invisible poisoning and stigmatizing effects.

A notorious governance crisis took place in association with the unfolding, the governmental authorities had loss of representativeness, and the capacity of broad responses necessary in the case was demonstrated as insufficient. Lack of transparency appeared on the side of the company as well as on the side of the public authorities.

The Seveso case fostered some relevant learning, shook the political atmosphere, and provided essential changes, the European Community improved regulation on disasters with the "Seveso" directive focusing different approaches on risk assessment with better public information dissemination as well as with public participation. In Italy, even the issue of abortion prohibition was brought to intense discussion within the supposed risk and fear of fetal malformation due to contamination. Answers not only for the accident but also for the different dimensions of consequences were required, then calling to responsibilities public agencies, political administrators, and regulators. The social and political crisis was recognized and had a proper role besides not having enough measurements, what showed the importance of recognizing uncertainties of several natures, as in the case of objective consequences in health and diseases, and the psychological, social, and political-related instabilities.

With much more direct impacts, the Bhopal disaster also characterized similar background of misinformation and extended consequences. At the early hours of December 3, 1984, the worst industrial accident registered occurred in the city of Bhopal, India, due to the leakage of methyl isocyanate (MIC) from the Union Carbide India Limited India, causing more than 2000 immediate deaths, although some estimated 200,000 injured, disabled, or subsequent deaths in the medium and long term. A very remarkable picture of pervasive ignorance was denoted by the ongoing aftermath of the disaster and the methods and doubts in providing relief to the victims. A succession of indecisions and misunderstandings established because of lack of information about the contaminant as well as its consequences of severe exposure to humans. The unpreparedness on behalf of the company, the authorities, doctors, nurses, police, fire-fighters, and other emergency response units showed a relation with insufficient scientific knowledge and absence of any previous risk communication (Jasanoff 1988).

The most affected victims of this accident were Muslims and Hindus living in conditions of social vulnerability in a peripheral neighborhood around the industrial plant. For the immediate victims, the contamination came causing discomfort, difficulty in breathing, burning eyes, and temporary blindness. Some of the survivors related that those with conditions tried to leave the proximity of the plant but without any information about the circumstances, causes, or possible damages. Many years after the accident, affected people are still suffering consequences or living with sequels. Some psychological implications happen to be overshadowed among the survivors, even in case of very severe unfolding, like mental disorders and suicide. The affected are still victimized by the continued disaster, which can be realized through the ongoing consequences, the insufficient justice stances, and weak attribution of the blame on the responsible, as well as through the negligence of subjective and intersubjective developments. Besides the acute impact of the accident, there was an implicit and different form of violence, one which is not impressive and instantaneous, but gradual and cumulative (Martins 2016).

The year 1984 was unfortunate in terms of chemical industrial accidents. Besides Bhopal, two other very significant incidents occurred: In San Juan Ixhuatepec in México, a leakage of liquid petroleum gas (LPG) brought about explosions destroying the facility of the company Petroleos Mexicanos (PEMEX) causing 550 deaths; in Cubatão, Brazil, an impoverished community of hundreds of stilt houses on a mangrove named Vila Socó was burned down due to leakage of 700,000 L of gasoline that came from the explosion of a pipeline network of the Brazilian oil company Petrobrás, killing more than 500 people. These three dramatic accidents had many things in common, like occurring in late-developing countries characterized by indebtedness and transference of activities potentially harmful for the environment and the public health in the sense of the second half-century context of political ecology (de Freitas et al. 1995). The standard background also conjoined poor, fast, and unplanned urbanization associated with industrialization as well as lack of environmental control and own legislation and competences. In the three cases, the majority of the affected were poor people settled in the urban industrial periphery coping with lack of social investments, water and sanitation, and health care, which characterizes the intensification of vulnerability and risks.

Abyssal asymmetries can be verified in such similar contexts. The first one that is very evident consists of the social exclusion and the socio-environmental vulnerability of poor people living in industrial peripheries. It is worthy to note again the parallel of social and cognitive exclusion, the last being not so evident but also fundamentally regarding the amplification of systemic consequences, and even with possible association with desirable preventive measures. For example, in the case of Bhopal, some previous signals of the risk of the accident were registered. Otherwise, the circumstances remained under the control of technical experts and managers, making no preventive adjustments. As Jasanoff (1988, p. 1118) stated: "*even unskilled workers could have been forewarned that a small amount of water accidentally released into the MIC tank could set off a reaction endangering thousands of lives*." In this sense, the right to know appears as something necessary and suitable to contribute to risk reduction, as well as it must break a paradigm of the concentration of knowledge among those who have domain and expertise.

Of course, these accidents brought opportunities of institutional learnings, legislation, and new practices, as the European regulation based on Seveso case. Moreover, the Bhopal accident and particular weaknesses, for instance, influenced positively significant legislative, academic, and industrial changes on safety, helping to save lives even in the United States (Willey et al. 2005), and supposedly in other countries. Moreover, the question that remains is as follows: On the background of potential disasters, is there a possibility for symmetrical dialog among companies, government, and society?

Although there are many current guidelines in order to boost the broad involvement of stakeholders in more sophisticated and fair structures of risk governance, there is deep and traditional conditioning behind the asymmetries, sharing on one side those forces that push forward the causal chains of hazard and vulnerabilities and on the other side those who have to carry the burden of risk, systemic consequences, death, and disease. Behind the critical conditions of vulnerability are common to find projects that can be much committed to economic development than with the complexity of the different layers of sustainability, mainly related to environmental awareness and social justice as to consider iniquities and potential damage to peoples' health. The Bhopal case, for example, was referred to a search for increasing agricultural production to reduce anger in India, and this motivation was the base for the Union Carbide establishment, as to produce chemical defensives for a green revolution. But at that time, there were no restrictions or preparedness to deal with possible side effects, risks, and consequences (Martins 2016).

Across the division of the different hemispheres, the domain of hegemonic knowledge represented by science and technology resources seems to make sense to demonstrate imbalance of power that is fundamental to the scenario of cognitive exclusion. Such a disparity can be encountered through the verification that there is no proper translation among different forms of knowledge, that is, the scientific and technological knowledge has no realistic possibility for direct interaction with common sense and laypeople.

In fact, this is a matter of a rigid border between the two hemispheres of the same system, the one that appears in its relation of proximity and interdependency on a threshold of a disaster, then denouncing the humiliating disproportionality among responsible and victims. This rigid border started to be built with the modernity myth of scientific and unshakable truth, and then kept increasing by other overwhelming forms of knowledge and gained notorious magnitude with the twentieth-century process of power and wealth concentration, also associated with the fluidity of capital in search for possibilities of improving profit.

As the concentration of power and wealth can be related to the capacity of a domain on science, this conjuncture engenders in oppressive contexts associating socio-environmental vulnerabilities alongside the cognitive exclusion. The borders then defined to keep poor people without conditions of living in safety as well as to make them as prisoners without a chance to have communication. In other words, people's concerns, perceptions, values, and understanding about risks have no admissibility in the dominant structure of knowledge and decision-making. Maybe there are many remarkable evolutions in terms of better communication of risk that must be much more than a method to spread information from the side of hegemonic knowledge. Anyhow, I consider the still persistent challenge to promote legitimate dialogical interactions.

The characteristic of cognitive exclusion as an aggravating factor is not particular of disasters in developing countries. The 2011 Fukushima triple disaster of earthquake, tsunami, and melt-down accident of nuclear power plants posed critical consequences in Japan, dividing society and techno-science through a harsh conflict on uncertainties about possible massive health consequences, generalized fear, and mistrust on technology. Many unresolved questions have been raised associating risks of radioactive contamination and health, like the daunting growth of thyroid cancer even among children, and suspicions of incidence of other diseases, disorders, or physical dysfunctions due to the consumption of vegetables and fish produced in some areas influenced by the disaster.

As Japanese people considered themselves as an advanced and modern nation, the Fukushima disaster was very traumatic for their psyche, making an association with the Chernobyl disaster in the then Soviet Union. In this case, the gaps regarding knowledge democracy appeared in the process of communication of potential effects and in the difficulties to assimilate uncertainties that were challenging. The burden of doubt came into fear and relevant psychological threats to the whole society. This relation of the impact of the event on the public opinion and related controversies also appeared with the turnover on the former trust in the technological superiority, changing to 70% of people's rejection on nuclear power in 2016. Otherwise, in this same year, due to other historical and geopolitical factors, Japanese people supported a conservative government that restored the nuclear industry again, resulting in a peculiar twisted situation (Tsukahara 2017).

Whether the events post-disaster are clear concerning the relation of cognitive exclusion and systemic consequences and oversights, there are also relevant points to remark in the sense of the lack of dialogical interactions with society related to the previous circumstances of a disaster. Then, it becomes necessary to argue on the relevance of such cognitive rupture sharing social actors by knowledge and power as elements of the causality of man-made disasters. Thus, the mining disaster of Mariana in Minas Gerais State, Brazil, brings some relevant reflections. In November 2015, a sizeable mine-tailing dam named Fundão, owned by Samarco Corporation, collapsed, causing a massive wave of toxic mud downstream the Doce River, killing 20 people, reaching the Atlantic Ocean and causing environmental, socioeconomic, and public health damages. The risks around the Samarco's dam seemed to be underestimated (Garcia et al. 2017), and the effects on health as well tend to be restricted to those causalities strictly related to the accident. But, the consequences went far through systemic interactions widening territorial and time scales causing a variety of negative influences on health through ecological imbalances and communicable diseases; respiratory, ophthalmologic, and skin problems; several symptoms, and behavioral and psychological disorders (Vormittag et al. 2018).

The local population and social scientists were concerned about the rupture of the dam, and this is what ultimately happened (Valencio 2016). Maybe every person living in a risk area influence by a dam can have this same perception and fear. Unfortunately, the people from Bento Rodrigues, the most affected location in Mariana, were right in their suspicions. However, it is remarkable that conventionally, as in this case, people living at risk as well as their perceptions, understandings, and knowings are not considered in the process of risk evaluation.

One evidence of the misconnection between the responsible company and the people at risk was that Bento Rodrigues dwellers were advertised about the tragedy by known persons that worked for third-party companies contracted by Samarco. Statements collected from affected people showed that there were no contingency plans involving the communities at risk, and this omission decayed on the company liability as well as on public authorities (Freitas et al. 2016). Furthermore, other previous stakes in dispute showed disproportionality in the relations of the company with the society. Among these stakes, there were: expansion of the productive scale even with some appointments on the risks of instability of the dam; consequent augmentation of mineral refuse disposition without interest on technological alternatives to reduce the disposal; elevation of the number of labor accidents; increase of water demand in detriment of scarcity posed to human water supply; and general orientation to a model of natural resources exportation prevailing over local social needs and ecosystem limits (Wanderley et al. 2016).

A few hours before the dam collapsed, some employees of the company related that earth tremors were coming from the dam, but they were asked to go back to work because it was something "normal." A variety of narratives like this are compiled through an extensive survey on media production made by Caldas (2017), showing the plurality of views on the accident as well as the inherent silencing and omissions that occurred previously and subsequently of this huge environmental disaster. But one very relevant thing to check throughout this extensive amount of data is that within asymmetrical relationships, the company and the authorities ignored not only the risk but also the people at risk and their capacities, perceptions, fears, desires, and needs. The local people's forms of knowledge on the possibility of a disaster and their understandings on how to proceed were something entirely disregarded. Maybe the main force to keep these divisions among authorities, company, and society is related to the strong economic dependence of the region as well as to the importance of the number of jobs provided by Samarco to the small and poor Mariana County. Anyhow, the negligence on local people's cognition seems to play a convenience part in the process of territorial dispossession of the supremacy of economic exploitation.

Concerning substantial relevance of communication systems on the disaster, Manoj and Baker (2007) stress three challenging categories which are technological, sociological, and organizational: First, the assets of technology that of course are not enough without strategies and advances in the other two categories. The sociological category strongly relies on the need of common languages and suitable translations to communicate with people at risk. Finally, the organizational category has something essential to account for regarding the hierarchical structures and some tendencies to have obstacles in communication. In the Samarco case, for instance, it seems that the fears of residents, as well as the suspicions of employees of low level on hierarchy, were far to be considered as relevant in making changes, producing warnings, or to be part of contingency plans.

Companies and governments can be responsible for many aspects of such a complex tissue of vulnerabilities, oppression, and risks, but they also have to learn that their supremacy in the domain of knowledge, the capacity of decision, and the legal domain is something that isolates lay people in a profound condition of asymmetry. Then, those institutions also have to be involved with people at risk and also must be keen to learn. In fact, this process of involving different and even antagonistic social actors must be stimulated to be a reflexive process of social learning (Wals 2007; Jacobi 2015; Xavier et al. 2018).

In summary, there is a need for dissuading the oppression to promote more symmetrical interactions through mutual learning. This process of learning must be oriented to liberation, and this precious idea must be applied to those who have been oppressed as well as to those who are corroborating to the scenario of oppression. Then, lay people who live at risk must be stimulated to a process of reflections since the perception of their importance in such socio-ecological systems, as they have their histories and lives, their knowings and doings, their relevance as workers or consumers as well as their rights. Those who classically constitute the oppressive scenarios must recognize that the subjectivities and intersubjectivities of people at risk can be fundamental in contingency plans, but besides, their values, perceptions, beliefs, and knowledge are significative constituents in the prevention as well as in the process of recovery from any possible disaster. That is a pathway to recognizing the need for a knowledge democracy, which is essential for fair and systemic approaches to reducing risks and improving resilience.

Just in the week I was writing this section, in January 2019, unfortunate and shameful news came about the collapse of another mining dam also in the State of Minas Gerais, Brazil. This time, in a same type of tailing dam, the amount of mud was significantly less, but the immediate consequences were much worse, indicating hundreds of deaths and missing persons. The Brumadinho disaster occurred on a dam belonging to Vale, a huge mining company in Brazil. Indeed, Vale and the Anglo-Australian BHP Billiton are the owners of Samarco, responsible for the 2015 accident in Mariana. The amount of first information received through media indicated some very comparable similarities, but of course, further investigation were necessary to bring more confident information. Anyhow, it seems to make the reproduction of the same wicked relations among different social actors, the victims being dispossessed of voices.

In this sense, we can consider that there is a real oppressive structure, and people at risk as residents and employees remain enclosed in such a frame. Some barriers to keep them disadvantaged are the lack of domain on scientific, technological, and legal aspects; the general disregard on common sense knowledge; the missing public power; and the overestimation of the economic extent on other dimensions of sustainability, that is, social and ecological.

The disproportionality of consequences and stakes is terrifying in such disasters. Large enterprises such as mining are to be considered to have the possibility of risk in terms of investments and perspectives of outcomes. Many factors seem to condition profit or financial losses, like the technological and logistic challenges, the commodities price variance, the risk of accidents, liabilities on environmental degradation, or loss of human lives as most critical adversities. In the tailing dam stewardship, there is a trend of the pressure of international price variance on the reduction of risk mitigation measures in order to keep high profitability. Then the cyclical process of price drop corroborates with the hypotheses of the increased frequency of tailing dam incidents. In such analysis, the fall in the last supercycle of commodities in 2013 onward tend to have the Mariana disaster as an icon (Davies and Martin 2009; Wanderley et al. 2016), but now recently adding also Brumadinho.

Tailing dam accidents as other human-made disaster have the property of uncertainty. Of course, there are procedures and safety standards as well as inspection and monitoring to make possible operation within the safety margin. However, some surprising factors or pressures can interplay with the conditioning of risk and uncertainties. In this sense, these accidents can be considered as post-normal problems, and as much as the level of uncertainty grows pushed by some pressures like price variance and improper practices and omissions, the more related stakes are overpassed. In this sense, there is the realization of injustice among two different groups of stakeholders, on one side, those associated with the enterprise, the investors, and on the other side people at risk. The first group is at risk of losing money, and the last are people who live in the area with the possibility of severe consequences, at risk of losing lives, territories, jobs, families, and hope.

Of course, companies are not something to be understood just as perverse, but it is necessary to realize that there are conflicts and disproportional relationships interplaying with uncertainties and risk. In Mariana, for example, as well as in Brumadinho, the jobs offered by mining companies were essential, and so the role of mining activity is enormous in the economic context at the local level and also for the state of Minas Gerais, and the whole countries' economy. So the relationship between the company and people at risk seem to be very confusing. People who live close to the dam can be at a high level of risk, but they can be wholly dependent on the mining economic activity. Some workers indeed can be in different hierarchical positions, those at the bottom have no voice, and those at the top as engineers and managers can have the possibility to decide on better safety practices or to denounce fails and inappropriate behaviors. However, they can be involved in the pressure for substantial outcomes and also as engineers and managers working for the company they are potential victims of disaster! This paradoxical background shows the duality in which there is an oppressor in the oppressed, and so, the need for liberation must be employing dialogical interactions, reciprocal learning, and consideration of different and pertinent views of the context. Also, it is convenient to recognize a tendency in which the oppressed can become the oppressors (Freire 2000), so in the case of economical and occupational dependencies, those who are living in immediate risk but working for the companies can adopt a posture to push down the activities, relativizing risks and enforcing others to accept vulnerability.

Cognitive exclusion is not only a matter of injustice. Indeed, I argue that those anti-dialogical implications and contexts are something to engender unsustainability, facilitating technological disasters, or contributing to extended consequences and system failures. Within disaster conditionings, cognitive exclusion can be considered as something to trigger significative erosion in the social relationships and in the interdependencies necessary to support those socio-ecological systems, then making an intrinsic role that can be related to causalities of disasters as well as to the unfolding and intensification of damages. In this sense, the so-called social amplification process shows this possibility of worsening critic events through the combination of social phenomena, being prone to blending situations in which risk communication is not suitable for those people at risk, unleashing misinformation and aggravating perspectives of consequences.

Actually, deep disparities are much known as the background of such accidents. However, as many authors and even public policies can be claiming for broader participation of stakeholders for risk governance and better resilience, the division is still abyssal, and the question of cognitive exclusion is not something circumstantial; this is at the base of the structure of power and hegemonic knowledge. Moreover, such deep fragmentation of society can even be an opportunity for dispossession and predatory search for profit.

Disasters of cognitive exclusion can be then conceived, having in mind that the impossibility of dialogical interactions among different social actors plays a determinant role somewhat in the causalities of a disaster as much as in the respective worsening of systemic consequences. Then, framing new understandings and practices to promote knowledge democracy means fostering a challenging process of social struggle against many historical forms of violence, exclusion, and marginalization. However, it also relates to reducing risks and consequences through cognitive justice.

References

Bartram, J., & Cairncross, S. (2010). Hygiene, sanitation, and water: Forgotten foundations of health. *PLoS Medicine, 7*, e1000367.

Bauman, Z. (1999). *Modernidade e ambivalência*. Rio de Janeiro: Zahar.

Benessia, A., & De Marchi, B. (2017). When the earth shakes… and science with it. The management and communication of uncertainty in the L'Aquila earthquake. *Futures, 91*, 35–45.

Berkes, F., Colding, J., & Folke, C. (2000). Rediscovery of traditional ecological knowledge as adaptive management. *Ecological Applications, 10*, 1251–1262.

Brown, P. (1992). Popular epidemiology and toxic waste contamination: Lay and professional ways of knowing. *Journal of Health and Social Behavior, 33*, 267–281.

Brydon-Miller, M., Greenwood, D., & Maguire, P. (2003). *Why action research?* Thousand Oaks: Sage Publications.

Carrillo-Santisteve, P., & Lopalco, P. L. (2012). Measles still spreads in Europe: Who is responsible for the failure to vaccinate? *Clinical Microbiology and Infection, 18*, 50–56.

Christopher, S., Watts, V., McCormick, A. K. H. G., & Young, S. (2008). Building and maintaining trust in a community-based participatory research partnership. *American Journal of Public Health, 98*, 1398.

Caldas M das GC. (2017). *Vozes e silenciamento em Mariana: crime ou desastre ambiental*. 2nd ed. BCCL/Unicamp, Campinas.

Dankel, D. J., Vaage, N. S., & van der Sluijs, J. P. (2017). *Post-normal science in practice*. Amsterdam: Elsevier.

Davies, M., & Martin, T. (2009). Mining market cycles and tailings dam incidents. In 13th International Conference on Tailings and Mine Waste, Banff, AB. Retrieved from http://www.infomine.com/publications/docs/Davies2009.pdf

de Alvarenga, A., de Souza Alvarez, A., Sommerman, A., & Philippi, A., Jr. (2015). Capítulo 2 Interdisciplinaridade e transdisciplinaridade nas tramas da complexidade e desafios aos processos investigativos. In A. Philippi Jr. & V. Fernandes (Eds.), *Práticas da interdisciplinaridade no ensino e pesquisa* (pp. 37–89). Barueri: Manole.

de Freitas, C. M., de S. Porte, M. F., & Gomez, C. M. (1995). Acidentes químicos ampliados: um desafio para a saúde pública. *Revista de Saúde Pública, 29*, 503–514.

De Marchi, B., & Ravetz, J. R. (1999). Risk management and governance: a post-normal science approach. *Futures, 31*, 743–757.

de Sousa Santos, B. (2004). *A universidade no século XXI: para uma reforma democrática e emancipatória da universidade*. São Paulo: Cortez.

de Sousa Santos, B. (2007). Para além do pensamento abissal: das linhas globais a uma ecologia de saberes. *Novos estudos-CEBRAP, 79*, 71–94.

de Sousa Santos, B. (2009a). *Una epistemología del sur: la reinvención del conocimiento y la emancipación social*. México: CLACSO y Siglo XXI.

de Sousa Santos, B. (2009b). *Um discurso sobre as ciências* (6th ed.). São Paulo: Cortez.

de Toledo, R. F., & Giatti, L. L. (2014). Challenges to participation in action research. *Health Promotion International, 30*, 162–173.

de Toledo, R. F., Giatti, L. L., & Pelicioni, M. C. F. (2012). Mobilização Social em Saúde e Saneamento em Processo de Pesquisa-ação em uma Comunidade Indígena no Noroeste Amazônico. *Saúde e Sociedade, 21*, 206–218.

Folke, C., Carpenter, S. R., Walker, B., et al. (2010). Resilience thinking: Integrating resilience, adaptability and transformability. *Ecology and Society, 15*, 20.

Foucault, M. (1980). *Power/knowledge. Selected Interviews and Other Writings of Michel Foucault*. New York: Pantheon Books.

Freire, P. (2000). Pedagogy of the oppressed (M. B. Ramos, Trans.; D. Macedo, introduction). 30th anniversary ed. New York: The Continuum International Publishing Group Inc.

Freitas, M., Alves, E., Santo, M., & Portella, S. (2016). O desastre da Samarco/VALE/BHP: Análise crítica de alguns discursos, racionalidades e percepções. *Ciência e Cultura, 68*, 51–56.

Funtowicz, S. O., & Ravetz, J. R. (1993). Science for the post-normal age. *Futures, 25*, 739–755.

Garcia, L. C., Ribeiro, D. B., Oliveira Roque, F., et al. (2017). Brazil's worst mining disaster: Corporations must be compelled to pay the actual environmental costs. *Ecological Applications, 27*, 5–9.

Giatti, L. L. (2013). *Uma contribuição à ciência pós-normal: aplicações e desafios da ampliação da comunidade de pares em contextos socioambientais e de saúde*. São Paulo: Universidade de São Paulo.

Giatti, L. L. (2015). *O paradigma da ciência pós-normal: participação social na produção de saberes e na governança socioambiental e da saúde*. São Paulo: Annablume.

Giatti, L. L., Landin, R., & de Toledo, R. F. (2014). Aplicabilidade da ecologia de saberes em saúde e ambiente e sua permeabilidade na produção acadêmica. *Ciência & Saúde Coletiva, 19*, 4091–4102.

Giatti, L. L., Rocha, A. A., de Toledo, R. F., et al. (2007). Condições sanitárias e socioambientais em Iauaretê, área indígena em São Gabriel da Cachoeira, AM. *Ciência & Saúde Coletiva, 12*, 1711–1723. https://doi.org/10.1590/S1413-81232007000600032.

Gibbons, M. (1999). Science's new social contract with society. *Nature, 402*, C81.

Gibbons, M., Limoges, C., Nowotny, H., et al. (1994). *The new production of knowledge: The dynamics of science and research in contemporary societies*. Thousand Oaks: Sage.

Gluckman, P. (2014a). *Evidence based policy: A quixotic challenge. Address given at the invitation of the science policy research unit*. Brighton, UK: University of Sussex.

Gluckman, P. (2014b). The art of science advice to government. *Nature, 507*, 163–165.

Hall, B. (2015). Beyond epistemicide: Knowledge democracy and higher education. Available in: http://unescochair-cbrsr.org/unesco/wp-content/uploads/2015/09/Beyond_Epistemicide_final.pdf (accessed 14 September 2019).

Hansson, S. O. (2017). Science denial as a form of pseudoscience. *Studies in History and Philosophy of Science Part A, 63*, 39–47.

Hochman, G. (2011). Vacinação, varíola e uma cultura da imunização no Brasil. *Ciência & Saúde Coletiva, 16*, 375–386.

Hoffman, A. J. (2015). *How culture shapes the climate change debate*. Palo Alto: Stanford University Press.

Hulme, M. (2007). The appliance of science. *The Guardian, 14*, 9.

Israel, B. A., Schulz, A. J., Parker, E. A., & Becker, A. B. (2008). Critical issues in developing and following community-based participatory research principles. In M. Minkler & N. Wallerstein (Eds.), *Community-based participatory research for health* (pp. 47–62). San Francisco, CA: Jossey-Bass.

Jacobi, P. R. (2015). Meio ambiente, riscos e aprendizagem social. *Revista Cadernos de Pesquisa: Pensamento Educacional 10*:346–364.

Jacques, P. J., Dunlap, R. E., & Freeman, M. (2008). The organisation of denial: Conservative think tanks and environmental scepticism. *Environmental Politics, 17*, 349–385.

Jasanoff, S. (1988). The Bhopal disaster and the right to know. *Social Science & Medicine, 27*, 1113–1123.

Johnson, S. (2008). *O mapa fantasma*. Rio de Janeiro: Zahar.

Klinke, A., & Renn, O. (2012). Adaptive and integrative governance on risk and uncertainty. *Journal of Risk Research, 15*, 273–292.

Kuhn, T. A. (1992). *A estrutura das revoluções científicas*. Perspectiva: São Paulo.

Lang, D. J., Wiek, A., Bergmann, M., et al. (2012). Transdisciplinary research in sustainability science: Practice, principles, and challenges. *Sustainability Science, 7*, 25–43.

Leff, E. (2017). Power-knowledge relations in the field of political ecology. *Ambiente & Sociedade, 20*, 225–256.

Lewin, K. (1946). Action research and minority problems. *Journal of Social Issues, 2*, 34–46.

Linkov, I., Trump, B. D., Anklam, E., et al. (2018). Comparative, collaborative, and integrative risk governance for emerging technologies. *Environment Systems and Decisions, 38*, 170–176.

List, D. (2006). Action research cycles for multiple futures perspectives. *Futures, 38*, 673–684.

Lucero, J. E., Wright, K. E., & Reese, A. (2017). Trust development in CBPR partnerships. In N. Wallerstein, B. Duran, J. G. Oetzel, & M. Minkler (Eds.), *Community-based participatory research for health: Advancing social and health equity* (p. 61). Hoboken: Wiley.

Macaia, A. A. S., Takahashi, M. A. C., Maeda, S. T., et al. (2018). Laboratório de Mudança: uma metodologia formative, participative e sistêmica para criação e transformação de sistemas de atividade. In R. F. de Toledo et al. (Eds.), *Pesquisa Participativa em Saúde: Vertentes e Veredas*. São Paulo, Brasil: Instituto de Saúde.

Manoj, B. S., & Baker, A. H. (2007). Communication challenges in emergency response. *Communications of the ACM, 50*, 51–53.

Martins, B. S. (2016). Revisitando o desastre de Bhopal: os tempos da violência e as latitudes da memória. *Sociologias, 18*, 116–148.

Mayr, E. (2005). *Biologia, ciência única*. São Paulo: Editora Companhia das Letras.

Morin, E. (2010). *Ciência com consciência* (14th ed.). Bertrand: Rio de Janeiro.

Nederland, C., & Groupe, U. R. D. (2013). Reaching resilience: Handbook 2.0 for aid practitioners and policymakers in disaster risk reduction, climate change adaptation and poverty reduction. CARE Nederland.

Nowotny, H. (2004). The potential of transdisciplinarity. In H. Dunin-Woyseth & M. Nielsen (Eds.), *Discussing transdisciplinarity: Making professions and the new mode of knowledge production, the Nordic reader* (pp. 10–19). Oslo: Oslo School of Architecture.

Pachauri, R. K., Mayer, L., & Intergovernmental Panel on Climate Change (Eds.). (2015). *Climate change 2014: Synthesis report*. Geneva: Intergovernmental Panel on Climate Change.

Querol, M. A. P., Jackson Filho, J. M., & Cassandre, M. P. (2011). Change laboratory: uma proposta metodológica para pesquisa e desenvolvimento da Aprendizagem Organizacional. *Administração: Ensino e Pesquisa, 12*, 609–640.

Ravetz, J. (2004). The post-normal science of precaution. *Futures, 36*, 347–357.

Raynaut, C. (2011). *Interdisciplinaridade: mundo contemporâneo, complexidade e desafios à produção e à aplicação de conhecimentos. Interdisciplinaridade em ciência, tecnologia & inovação* (pp. 143–208). Barueri: Manole.

Renn, O. (2008). *Risk governance: Coping with uncertainty in a complex*. World London: Earthscan Ltd.

San Sebastián, M., & Hurtig, A. K. (2005). Oil development and health in the Amazon basin of Ecuador: The popular epidemiology process. *Social Science & Medicine, 60*, 799–807.
Schatzki, T. (2015). *Spaces of practices and of large social phenomena* (p. 24). Montreal: Espaces Temps.
Snow, J. (1999). Sobre a maneira de transmissão do cólera.
Strand, R. (2017). Post-normal science. In *Routledge Handbook of Ecological Economics* (pp. 288–298). Abingdon: Routledge.
Thiollent, M. (2011). *Metodologia da Pesquisa-Ação* (18th ed.). São Paulo: Cortez.
Tsukahara, T. (2017). Commentary: New currents in science: The challenge of quality, examining the discrepancies and incongruities between Japanese techno-scientific policy and the citizens' science movement in post-3/11 Japan. *Futures, 91*, 84–89.
Valencio, N. (2016). Elementos constitutivos de um desastre catastrófico: os problemas científicos por detrás dos contextos críticos. *Ciência e Cultura, 68*, 41–45.
Van den Hove, S. (2000). Participatory approaches to environmental policy-making: The European commission climate policy process as a case study. *Ecological Economics, 33*, 457–472.
Vormittag, E. D. M. P. A., Araujo, D., Oliveira, M. A. D., & Gleriano, J. S. (2018). Health evaluation of the Barra Longa population affected by the disaster in Mariana County. *Ambiente & Sociedade, 21*, e01222.
Walker, B., Holling, C. S., Carpenter, S. R., & Kinzig, A. (2004). Resilience, adaptability and transformability in social–ecological systems. *Ecology and Society, 9*, 5.
Wallerstein, N., & Duran, B. (2010). Community-based participatory research contributions to intervention research: the intersection of science and practice to improve health equity. *American Journal of Public Health, 100 Suppl 1*, S40–S46.
Wallerstein, N., & Duran, B. (2017). Theoretical, historical, and practice roots of CBPR. In N. Wallerstein, B. Duran, J. G. Oetzel, & M. Minkler (Eds.), *Community-based participatory research for health: Advancing social and health equity* (p. 17). Hoboken: Wiley.
Wallerstein, N., Giatti, L. L., Bógus, C. M., et al. (2017). Shared participatory research principles and methodologies: Perspectives from the USA and Brazil—45 years after Paulo Freire's "Pedagogy of the Oppressed". *Societies, 7*, 6.
Wals, A. E. (2007). *Social learning towards a sustainable world: Principles, perspectives, and praxis*. Wageningen: Wageningen Academic.
Wanderley, L. J., Mansur, M. S., Milanez, B., & Pinto, R. G. (2016). Desastre da Samarco/Vale/ BHP no Vale do Rio Doce: aspectos econômicos, políticos e socio ambientais. *Ciência e Cultura, 68*, 30–35.
Wildemeersch D (2007) Social learning revisited: Lessons learned from north and south. In Wildemeersch D, Wals AEJ Social learning towards a more sustainable world Wageningen University Press, Wageningen, 99–116.
Willey, R. J., Crowl, D. A., Lepkowski, W. (2005). The Bhopal tragedy: its influence on process and community safety as practiced in the United States. *Journal of loss prevention in the process industries 18*:365–374.
World Health Organization—WHO. (2018). *Europe observes a 4-fold increase in measles cases in 2017 compared to previous year* (p. 6). Geneva: World Health Organization.
Xavier, L. Y., Jacobi, P. R., Turra, A. (2018). On the advantages of working together: Social Learning and knowledge integration in the management of marine areas. *Marine Policy 88*:139–150.

Chapter 3
Participation and Sustainability

3.1 Beyond the Hegemonic Knowledge

Beyond hegemonic production, there is a broad variety of other kinds of knowledge that have always been associated with social practices and problem-solving. These much different forms of knowledge are necessary for everyday interactions with adversities and scarcities, as well as constituting primary determinants in imbricated causal relations and associated with several critical problems as those related to health, environment, and sustainability. Therefore, to promote a reasonable reflection on the perspective of the ecology of knowledge, it is necessary to illustrate some aspects and cases denoting the importance of the diversity of knowledge, then recognizing its relation with innovation throughout participatory approaches, in the sense of fostering interaction and co-creation of new, hybrid, and applicable knowledge.

Elementary concepts from natural sciences can contribute to understanding the role and importance of diversity in complex systems. Of course, this is not a stance in a reductionist point of view, even though the idea is approaching socio-ecological systems. Then fragmentations among nature and human systems would not be suitable, but it is worthy to note that there are some relevant analytical issues to consider from the perspective of natural sciences. As a starting point, some transcendent concepts can be applicable to different kinds of systems as well as to different organizational scales (Von Bertalanffy 1968). For instance, a significant contribution discussed here is the self-organization principle, which can be applicable to cells, organisms, or biological communities. Self-organization is related to the capacity to respond in the face of any change or disturbance, but also represents possibilities to find alternatives, demonstrating the plasticity of specific systems, organisms, or communities within the surrounding environment. It also concerns a constant search for balance with the environment and interactions with similar or others.

L. L. Giatti, *Participatory Research in the Post-Normal Age*,
https://doi.org/10.1007/978-3-030-27924-0_3

Therefore, based on assumptions from natural systems, biological diversity is indicated in correlation with an adaptive competence and resilience, that is to say, the more diversity exists in a system, the more this system can provide answers and alternatives to cope with changes, impacts, and disturbances. From the perspective of socio-ecological systems, the more the diversity the more alternatives a system can have to evolve to a better or desirable condition. In that way, it is remarkable to recognize this attribute: "desirable," because it is inherent to the subjectivity of socio-ecological systems.

In the book *The Quark and the Jaguar* Gell-Mann (1995) examines exciting aspects from the simple to the complex and then makes a productive contribution in a correlation between biodiversity and adaptability. For him, the complexity of an ecosystem can be associated with the amount of genetic information available from the diversity of species. In this sense, the genetic information has the property of a sort of algorithms as potentialities to adapt. Therefore, ecosystems richer in species means it is abundant with self-organizing alternatives. In complementary meaning, the more diverse, the more complex, and the more able to adapt or to have conditions in finding pathways to return to a previous system integrity in the face of disturbance—i.e., more resilient (Walker et al. 2004).

Dealing with natural systems isolated, there has been a background in which the degree of complexity can be considered ordinary. Applying to socio-ecological systems, the associated complexity is that one with emergent properties, where the subjectivity, intersubjectivity, communication, and language play a role of overlapping layers of expanded and intrinsic relations and possibilities of change. Anyhow the faculty of autonomy, self-organization, and coupling in the sense of collaborative relationships are also attributable to socio-ecological systems.

Organization, for instance, is a property inherent to living and can be related to the adaptive capacity as any cells, organisms, species, or communities can have a degree of plasticity to cope with environmental changes and disturbances. Self-organization is even obligatorily related to autonomy. Moreover, the plasticity in biological systems can have their basis in genetic and physiological characteristics, then making it possible for the system to establish or evolve in terms of its structure, which is related to the components and relations. Applying this to socio-ecological systems, it is worthy to outline Maturana and Varela's words (1992, p. 176): "*in an organism with a nervous system rich and vast as that of human beings, its realms of interaction open the way to new phenomena by allowing new dimensions of structural coupling. In human beings, this makes for language and self-consciousness*."

Special attention must be given to the capability of coupling, which can be interpreted as the process of collaborative building of new knowledge, or in other words an ecology of knowledge, then providing new system structures and enhancing the organizational capacities through collaborative interactions. This supposition can contribute to previous ideas from the beginning of the twentieth century (Kropotkin 2012), bringing a counterpoint to the assumption of Darwin and Wallace that struggle for existence is the central factor for evolution. In this sense, the very remarkable point is that mutual aid and collaboration among communities and species, or human beings, can represent evolution and adaptability much more than, sometimes, the struggle for existence. That is a point for a substantial philosophical, biological, and sociological discussion, even nowadays within the mindset of competitiveness as a key value in human society. Human cooperation has been intrinsic to our evolutionary dynamics as a supremely social species, and current research on this has demonstrated a cornerstone on the relevance and potentiality of mutual aid for collective outcomes. Such contemporary understanding has helped to surpass the conundrum of the opposing competition for natural selection. Anyhow, cooperation among humans occurs in a broad range of situations and can be associated and powered by learning and culture (Rand and Nowak 2013).

Structural coupling is here considered as the potential of making possible interactions to combine biological, material, and cognitive diversities to create new and hybrid solutions, also fostering knowledge democracy. In that way, a genuine process of cooperation and expansion of responsiveness. From given preexistent diversity in a system, the property of structural coupling can represent something to boost new diversities as possible interactions and alternatives, then adding robustness to system structures. In such a perspective, the systems involving human societies can have more possibilities of creating alternatives, but also, can create new situations and new developments, environments, and processes.

The issue of studying the self-organizing properties of a socio-ecological system can be challenging, but entirely necessary to find significant explanations and causal determinants in these interplaying networks of knowings, doings, values, perceptions, and interests, among other conditioning. For example, a superficial point of view on the organizational aspects of a slum can even result in prejudiced and reductionist views. On the other hand, a dedicated and detailed ethnographic study on a slum can show that even in such precarious urban community it is possible to identify and understand a profusion of alternatives, associated with social practices created, established, and reproduced by people. This plurality of social practices, entirely related to local knowledge, are as well responses to the in-depth scenarios of contingencies and vulnerabilities, and sometimes these alternatives can be very indicative of pertinence towards the context of globalization as reproducing pressures on those vulnerable urban peripheries (Magnani 2002).

Lack of fundamental resources like food, energy and water, inexistence of sanitation, urban violence, precarious access to health care, and general insufficiency of public policies are some relevant constraints in impoverished urban peripheries. These constraints are part of material conditionings that embed the co-creation of doings and knowings, or in other words, the correspondent social practices and common sense knowledge. In this perspective, social life is an inherent part of practice-arrangement bundles where the social phenomenon takes place, then giving the attribute of central importance to the social practices and their intermediations within other practices even in different scales like from the local to global and vice versa (Schatzki 2015).

However, the predominance of subjectivity, unpredictability, and ambivalence in such bundle of social practices seems to be something aggressive to the hegemonic knowledge production that continually searches for objectivity and truth within the modern dilemma and the positivist rationality. The mainstream problem-solving tendency with regard to science–policy interactions has shown the expectation of implementing full-scale solutions for the social problems, and maybe this is much more related to industrial scaling, ignoring the diversity of interactions among the society (Bauman 1999). Massification as a pattern tends to diminish and conceal the diversity of ideas, possibilities, and practices. Trying to impose "mechanic" and top-down solutions into a variety of contexts seems to give support to what Santos (Santos 2009b; Santos et al. 2016) calls a monoculture of knowledge. Thus, it can unleash epistemicide and a sociology of absences, when the Western thinking discredits and wastes all of the world's historical social experience, that, indeed, is much more extensive and varied than the scientific tradition.

Much possible innovation can come from other rationalities. Thus alternative systems of production, solidary economy, legal pluralism, cultural citizenship, and alternative ownership rights must be contemplated as opportunities to encourage what Santos proposes as a sociology of emergencies with the objective of strengthening different epistemologies with authentic hope from those which are classically separated by abyssal lines.

From the urban anthropology point of view (Magnani 2002), a poor urban community, for instance, can benefit from diversity, that instead of being fragmented multiculturalism, represents systems of exchanges, unimaginable partnerships, innovative forms of cooperation, initiatives, and experiences of different nuances. In a peripheral urban community, a diversity to sum and make a myriad of coupling can be related to ethnic or regional identities, cultural preferences, creeds, sexual orientation, groups oriented on several political directions, and minorities or social groups marked by exclusion. It is worthy to recognize in this sense that top universities around the world have fostered diversity among their student and educational boards. However, as making more innovative indoor environments, it does not make legitimate dialogical interactions with the rage of diverse knowledges outside the academics. Isolated from broad interactions with the whole society, diversity in the universities can make difference and competitiveness, but not necessarily promote cognitive justice and authentic social inclusion.

The diversity of socio-ecological systems attracts interest. With respect to new arrangements and solutions, sometimes creating opportunities to manage scarce resources from the local level, diversity, and structural coupling are supposed to make possible intelligible links with the global main ecological concerns, as the climate change dynamics and the planetary boundaries regarding the exhaustion of essential material inputs, energy, water resources, and the drastic reduction of biodiversity (Rockström et al. 2009; Steffen et al. 2015). The number of innovative alternatives offered through ecology of knowledge also can bring closer the matter of scarcity and unsustainability to deal with the determinants of health, then pushing forward joined alternatives for the quality of life as reducing risks of diseases, suffering, and avoidable early deaths. The insight is to conceive ecology of knowledge instead of monoculture, and this can be applied making use and disclosing associations with biodiversity and epistemic diversity as well as to recognize the relevance of a diversity of social practices and knowings through necessary and equitable interactions.

3.2 Other Knowledges and Routes to Sustainability

Regarding communities in vulnerable conditions and facing sorts of scarcities, it is also possible to find many exciting learnings from rural and indigenous societies. As to observe environmental constraints, tropical ecosystems can provide some notable examples. Amazon biome, for instance, calls some representations of life in abundance and consequently plenty of food and resources. Otherwise, the Blackwater ecosystems as the Upper Rio Negro at Northwest Amazon between Colombia, Venezuela, and Brazil, represent challenging extremely nutrient-poor environments, mainly concerning protein availability.

In such hard ecological conditions, Moran (1991) relates a variety of human-adaptive strategies for surviving, forging a cultural aspects strait associated with the surrounding scarcity. Within these strategies, the development of forms of exchange and specialization among different ethnic groups; hierarchical control over the more productive places for fishing; population disposition in tiny settlements at considerable distances from each other; and a strong dependence on bitter manioc to provide the daily calorie needs.

Detailing on those adaptive practices can even exhibit arrangements very surprising that through mythical explanations contribute to regulate and manage the access to resources. In this regard, Tukano people, one of the ethnic groups that occupy the region probably for more than 1000 years, developed a very sophisticated system of sharing and controlling the access to hunting resources. For Tukano people, the bigger an animal is, the more it has a concentration of the kind of "energy" that will be absorbed by someone who eats its meat. The practical concern in this sense is that if someone overeats meat, the accumulation of such "energy" can make the person vulnerable to the forest entities, bringing the risk of suffering an accident or attack, having the canoe turned in the river, or even killed by a snake bite. What happens then is a discipline not only of sparingly eating but sharing the food, mainly when someone hunts a big animal. This is basic for collective surviving, as the same contributes to regulating hunting stock. Somehow, the practice is based on their cultural understanding of their environment and with their means of creating explanations that effectively work to the tenuous balance among the ecosystem capacity to provide protein and their communal needs (Hildebrand and Bunyard 1993).

I had a great life experience as working for IBAMA (Brazilian Institute of Environment and Natural Resources) during one and a half years (2003–2004) in the Upper Rio Negro, precisely headquartered in São Gabriel da Cachoeira County, a small city that acts as the capital city of the enormous territory of the Blackwater in Brazilian Northwestern Amazon. There I had the opportunity to visit many indigenous communities to know something about their dynamics, resources, scarcities, and challenges. One of the more dramatic problems for those people was the access to health care due to the very vast territory with more than four hundred communities of different sizes. In the health assistance model, health care teams with a doctor used to travel by boat for several days to reach the communities along the rivers of the Rio Negro basin, like Waupés, Içana, and others. One of the most prominent health problems was the high prevalence of tuberculosis among the indigenous, including occurrence of antibiotic-resistant strains. So when a doctor diagnosed a tuberculosis case in a small community, he or she had to provide medicines for that patient for an extended period, like 1 month. The patient received the medicine and instructions on how to administer the same. Afterwards, when the doctor came back to the community, it appeared that the patient was worse, and the investigation on the circumstances was shocking: the patient had distributed the pills for all the people in the community. Well, for them, medicine is a scarce resource, and their culture seems to have dictated on how to proceed.

Besides the cultural shock, this is a situation that shows both sides: the traditional knowledge, values, and practices are essential for their centuries-old ways of coping with ecological scarcities; on the other side, applying recommendations or implementing solutions that do not consider the cultural background can result in a grave disappointment. Moreover, this critical unfolding also demonstrates the lack of preparedness of the health care teams to deal with these complex contexts of health determinants.

The case of an indigenous community in Amazon suits very well to the point of view grounded classically in the primary assumption of the world divided into colonies and metropolis. Anyhow, the discrepant values, practices, and knowledges, even those structured through peculiar genealogies, call attention and help us to understand that there are fundamental differences between common sense and hegemonic scientific thinking. Moreover, those differences are argued to be determinant in association with sustainability and health. However, the cartography of contradictions nowadays is not so clearly delimitated, and the discrepancy between knowledges as well as the cognitive exclusion can be occurring everywhere, even in urban contexts of the global North (De Sousa Santos 2007). What is really important to stress is that the lack of knowledge democracy is not only a question related to injustice but is also related to sustainability. Thus, cognitive inclusion through the participation of stakeholders and dialogical interactions means at finding the more sophisticated and efficient alternatives to deal with complex issues and to deliver alternatives able to adapt to the sociocultural contexts.

For example, the issue of access to health sometimes is related to vulnerability components instead of the lack of health services. Furthermore, regarding public policies, the insufficient access to health care can also be related much more to inadequacies than to the absence of specific policies. In North Belfast, Ireland, a rapid participatory appraisal (Lazenbatt et al. 2001) was applied to define health and social needs of people of a deprived area, in order to improve access to primary health care. Within this initiative, and thanks to the involvement of local dwellers, it was realized that much important health and social needs could not be met by health services provision alone. The interactive process also made possible a direct transfer of skills and information to local women that became able to secure resources for the community and helped to build and share important narratives on the factors that were related to health care access, like unmet needs causing distrust among the public. This approach helped to emerge hidden determinants that became the basis for community and for health professionals to address efficient alternatives, valuing local knowings and perceptions. Another aspect is that the holistic and collaborative appraisal also helped to bring broader understandings on the high local dependence on the prescription of drugs such as antidepressants that appeared as reinforcing addictive behaviors among women in order to cope with stress and the surrounding features of poverty and vulnerability.

In Alberta, Canada, one more enriching experience shows the feasibility of collaborative knowledge and action. A project to stimulate relationships among local stakeholders, university, and government aimed at improving the health of the community and gathering and applying evidence to influence values and to change environments (Raine et al. 2010). The focus was on obesity and chronic diseases, and the intervention framework combined collaborative work diagnosis and classification of the environment by types. The typology considered physical, economic, political, and socio-cultural aspects that could be relevant for health promotion, followed by finding some perspectives of changes through expanding communitarian gardening; fostering active transportation; facilitating free access to leisure facilities; and development of a social enterprise to address food insecurity. This project also allowed new and distinguished understandings, contributing to local capacity building and the setting up off original establishing effectiveness for population health interventions.

In both experiences, in Belfast and in Alberta, the participatory approach was the process to engender the cognitive inclusion through successive dialog among common sense and the hegemonic knowledge, represented by researchers and health professionals. In Belfast, the interaction with the community was carried out through workshops, focus groups, and collaborative surveys within the communities. The participatory process among other results and perspective of actions suit to bring what the authors called "hidden troubles." In Alberta, a community-based participatory framework enabled the interaction, same as with successive tools. Also, this both participatory research and action experiences demonstrated that there is a need to fostering ongoing interactions and feedback, in a method destined to reach the objective of a real collaborative process, a legitimate and plural diagnosis, and a problem-solving targeting. That is the procedure to make possible interaction among a diversity of ideas, values, interests, and understandings as to impulse the ecology of knowledge building feasible alternatives.

Moreover, these participatory experiences also shed light on the relevance of cognitive elements from the community, not only as something fair to be taken into consideration, but a real basis for functional solutions and also in a standpoint in which the same approach that fosters cognitive inclusion additionally makes attainable the collaborative alternatives, and above all promotes dialogical reflection and social learning (Bawden et al. 2007).

Going back to the peculiar knowledge and behavior of the Tukano people, there is a great distance to be crossed to make possible collective knowledge and collaborative solutions to deal with sustainability and health issues. However, such a distance is not only pronounced because of the difference among the knowledges and their epistemic trajectories, there is also a relevant matter associated with a substantial concentration of power and consequent lack of trust, everything engendered in the substantive and historical process of domination from the surrounding "white" national society on those indigenous and ancestor communities. The relationship among those communities and the involving society dates to the colonial times and is still representative of prejudice and the continuous will to "integrate" the indigenous, as something to disregard the ancient knowledge and the successful practices of surviving in those environments with lack of essential resources like protein.

The typical relationship among surrounding society and indigenous people is still tendentious to the epistemicide, what is referred to as killing other knowledge systems. On the other hand, the perspective of searching for sustainability with integration and dialogical relationship is to acknowledge the importance of multiple knowledge systems, such as spiritual and land based. The strengthening of knowledge democracy can be based on frameworks arising from social movements and own marginalized knowledges and practices. The action of inclusion by means of participatory approaches represents to deepen in democracy through giving space to a legitimate struggle for a fairer and healthier world (Hall and Tandon 2017).

Furthermore, other contemporary criticisms and proposals also recognize the primary role of participation and stakeholder inclusion to cope with the global challenge of unsustainability. With regard to the ecosystem services framework, a recent argument of "nature's contribution to people" criticizes the failure to engage social sciences as well as local knowledges, values, and interests. Indeed, the challenging issue of being inclusive must be broadened enough to allow different strands of knowledge, representation of worldviews, interests, and values. Anyhow, this view encompasses an understanding of reciprocity towards common obligations shared by people and nature, as well as it remits to a coproduction of alternatives (Díaz et al. 2018).

For example, Brazil, a vast food producer and international exportation player, is strongly dependent on the ecosystem service pollination, which means a potential for production improvement as well as a warranty for national and international food security. However, pollination has been threatened by diverse factors as loss of habitat, climate change, environmental pollution, agrochemicals, invading species, and diseases (Wolowski et al. 2018). Then, accessing nature's contribution to people concerning pollination as a collaborative trial should involve indigenous people or other rural residents as knowledge holders, then finding common alternatives as to define practices of care like fostering pollinator nesting resources. That is a scope of interaction and learning among nature and people, so it is important to stress that the unfolding should be understood through a plurality of cultural lens, requesting suitable opportunities for strengthening the social dimensions to deal with this delicate ecological issue.

In the ecological economics field, mainly at the sphere of scientific production in the journal with the same name, there is some appointment on evolution towards a post-normal science since the 1990s. However, the simple recognition of the nature of post-normal problems as those multifaceted and permeated by uncertainties in association with ecological ones is not enough to make real a new practice. A particular element in order to do convergence with post-normal science is the extended peer community, something to reach not only with recommendations but effectively with stakeholders' involvement as practicing collaboration in new forms of problem-solving. Then, it is required to create innovative approaches to characterize, communicate, and manage with scientific uncertainty, thus focusing the social reality at the scope of controversies and conflicts in the face of the erosion of trust among experts and nonexperts (Strand 2017).

Peterson et al. (2018) argue that the complex character of the coproduction of nature's contributions to people requires approaches to bridge and make respect on the integrity of different knowledge systems. That is a question on building practical knowledge for sustainability in a diverse world, weaving together collaborations involving knowledge mobilization, translation, negotiation, and application.

In such frame of necessary interactions, participatory research can be considered as compelling alternatives for knowledge democratization throughout ongoing processes of interaction. Therefore, in this case of indigenous people versus the tendency of marginalization, or even in closer situations like in urban contexts, the issue of trust building is a significant point to consider and to manage.

The conventional relationship of academic with other knowledge is based on lack of trust and oppression. Otherwise, the alternative of true dialogical and symmetrical collaborations requires sharing power. In fact, the lack of complete domain on a research or intervention process seems to be something terrifying to researchers. Scientists are classically applying methods in which they have control over variables, methods, and measurements. Otherwise, participatory research appears as entirely different because, at the beginning of any process, there is no perspective of progress without communitarian acceptance and involvement. This sharing of power is a transformation for researchers in their relationship with the object of study, but it is essential for reciprocity in the interaction. So, without a doubt, such a stance is needed for building and maintaining trust, as a central role in the success or failure of any project of this nature (Christopher et al. 2008; Lucero et al. 2017).

Trust! That is a highly sensitive point in dialogical processes. There must be a perspective of engagement and balanced collaboration and interaction in the participatory process. People from the communities, classically marginalized for their way of knowing, must encounter means to value their point-of-view, their experiences, and understandings. In sum, the perspective of cognitive inclusion has association with a cultural action based on the potentialities of the social entity to be involved. This is very basic for trust building, and it is at the core of a process of more symmetrical interactions, entirely necessary to allow reciprocity in learning and teaching. So the researchers must be humble, and lay people must have the opportunity to reflect on their perspectives to consider themselves as relevant in the process (Freire 2000). There is supremacy to validate the capacity of any person to recognize himself or herself as a fundamental piece in a socio-ecological system. Indeed, in the Freirian assumptions, there are possibilities of transforming realities employing conscious practical action that can be related to the capacity of reading the world, something that naturally precedes the proficiency of reading the word or acquiring literacy (Freire 1985).

As I have argued in this chapter, the nature of organization runs within social groups and makes a myriad of alternatives. Otherwise, the abyssal lines established by the duality of worlds, one of the hegemonic knowledge and other of the marginalized, make the oppressive relationship. It's no surprise to conceive that there is a lack of trust in this context. The principle of autopoiesis (Maturana and Varela 1992) helps with some very remarkable understanding: autopoietic organization happens as a process which constantly defines any system or organism as a dynamic unity. When a system adapts itself, at the same time it turns into something different. In other words, there is no separation between producer and product.

Marginalized knowledges and practices are dynamic and continuously transformative, but the hegemonic knowledge still ignores them. So, it is tough to make possible the necessary the structural coupling between common sense, science, and decision-making that appropriates scientific discourses. In this sense, the insurmountable obstacle characterizes this oppressive circumstance: the lack of possibility to interact with the hegemonic knowledge ceases the skill of autopoiesis. Such dispossession can redefine marginalized social groups as those blocked to coupling with those who produce academic knowledge and/or with those who can appropriate the academic knowledge and have power for decision-making.

On the systemic perspective, any community or group is able to have a natural propensity to organize itself in dealing with other levels of organizations, as decision-making companies, to operate the ecology of knowledge and democratic protagonism. Otherwise, in analyzing the ruptures of knowledge and power, marginalization, and oppressive conjunctures, communities or groups are constrained of interacting and self-organizing (in the sense of autopoiesis). This process of segregation can happen in extremely differentiated contexts. For instance, an urban poor community becomes peripheral also by the lack of possibility to self-organize and interact with a policymaker due to anti-dialogical structures. As the same, medium class groups also become peripheral when they cannot interact with those who are using scientific discourse to decide on the application of new technology with risks that can be overshadowed, excluding those people at potential risk from the necessary debate on stakes and uncertainties.

Maybe it is a new face of oppression that arises in this late phase of our modernity, urging for correspondent action in producing renewed structures of dialogical reflection. That is because, when we analyze the current complex and emergent phenomena, classically excluded people, as well as those included (medium classes, people living in high-income societies), can be both excluded in terms of cognition. The Fukushima disaster brings a lesson in that direction, on the scenario of normality before the accident, everything seemed to work right, and there was no indication of cognitive exclusion. Suddenly, the disaster exposed its dimensions, and then oppression appeared with lack of preparedness, uncertain facts, and a severe governance crisis. Such a disruptive scenario of oppression can be seen as an unfolding of the previous alienation on the magnitude of hidden, unknown or ignored risks, in which the whole society had not dedicated enough effort to explore and discuss.

Other issues of our contemporary times with possible controversies and high stakes can make the same scenario of false normality, in which the societies accept a superficial discourse on risks versus benefits, and then, they also accept the promise of comfort, well-being, and economic development. Such characteristics can be identified in the controversies on the adoption of GMOs, or on the denial of anthropogenic causes of climate change when it threatens specific patterns of consumption. Such a condition of alienation and acceptance, when related to tragic unfolding, unveils people as oppressors of their own, in the case of the emergence of associated disasters and systemic negative consequences. In effect, both technological promises with the characteristic of post-normal problems and the digital inclusion represented by the potentialities of the internet do not seem to make great advantage for a reflexive society. Such context is problematic when conforming standardization of views and inertia. On the other side, there would be necessary to dialog on the complex scenarios to promote and make interactions of a diversity of ideas, instead of a monoculture of knowledge.

In the very attractive book *Sapiens: A Brief History of Humankind*, Harari (2016) presents a remarkable counterpoint to the beginning of agriculture and related results to *Homo sapiens*' development. Since 70,000 years ago, with an acceptable theory demonstrating peculiar genetic changes in the inside connections of the brain, a substantial neurological development gave the opportunity to a cognitive revolution. This biological evolution came associated with communication abilities, the possibility of flexible cooperations, development of myths and narratives relevant for social organization, and extensive plasticity in terms of identifying alternatives for survival and acquisition of food. The climax in this sense seems to be the ancient hunter-gatherers, who probably were the most skilled people of the entire human history. Hunter-gatherers had knowledge and abilities that were more comprehensive, more in-depth, and more varied than other social groups like sedentary farmers. Surprisingly, those nomads had a much more comfortable itinerant life than any one of their successors, as well as a diverse and plentiful diet. Agriculture then came to make profound changes in human behavior as well as reducing the diversity of diets, lack of safety leading to possible invasions and, above all, reduced the scope of cognitive capacities significantly, giving place to specialization into a short variety of abilities. Accordingly, Harari even states that plants domesticated humans and not the opposite, simplifying their routines and cognitive capacities.

These are quite instigating assumptions, and maybe it can make us reflect on the historical revolutions and their role concerning the potentialities of our species. Anyhow, the contemporary revolution of communication through the internet and the use of smartphones and social networking will make new conditioning to our abilities. Otherwise, it will probably pose some unexpected collateral effects, as to reduce reflexivity and increase intolerance, reducing peoples' conversations only among those with the same assumptions and then bringing other forms of social erosion or even giving support to tyranny (Snyder 2017). There will be necessarily much more evidence and study on the current internet-related repercussions. Anyhow, the consequence of the isolation of common sense and marginalized knowledge seems to be something with a definite possibility to confine possibilities of innovative structural coupling, and maybe the current digital dynamics can perform a role in that direction.

Back to the Tukano people and other ethnic groups from the upper Rio Negro, they can be understood as demonstrating essential lessons about self-organization and human cooperation. They work collaboratively, involving different groups to manage the scarce resources of the environment, sharing knowledges, goods, and territories. In this sense, they demonstrate more intent in collective interest and survival than in mere individualism or competition (Moran 1991). Such background can corroborate with the hypothesis of Kropotkin (2012), that cooperation can be more relevant than competition in certain circumstances. Moreover, other ethnographic examples can encompass a considerable amount of examples of structural coupling through individual or group cooperation, and this can be verified in urban slums like with the dynamics or reciprocities, solidarity, and social practices (Magnani 2002). Also, collective experiences of vulnerable people trigger city making in peripheries where public power is absent, exhibiting a sort of merge of knowledge that also reflects the emergence of collective imagination and action to solve local urban demands (Holston 2009).

Fostering ecology of knowledge is not only a question of cognitive justice but also an obvious alternative for collaboration and a pathway to permeate the barriers that divide the world into academic and nonacademic knowledge holders—making possible dialogical interactions among marginalized, hegemonic knowledge, and decision-making that must provide another level of interactions, innovations, and possibilities for transitions to sustainability. Ecologizing knowledge and promoting dialogical reflections also relate to uncover or foresee emergent scenarios in which societies can be the oppressors of their own, due to the magnitude and systemic unfolding of emergent crises and side effects of technological innovation.

Ecology of knowledge is creative in the sense of optimizing the possibility of merging diversities of ideas and practices into unprecedented bundles of achievable adaptive alternatives. That is to allow and foster multi-stakeholder interactions pursuing common concerns about how the world and the people must be treated to democratically target sustainability (Bawden et al. 2007). It means at pushing forward a new constellation of alternatives, then bringing a diversity of legitimate knowings, social practices to cope with a diverse world with a plurality of scarcities and contradictions. Furthermore, the ecology of knowledge is a clamor for bringing back a whole competency of interacting, once the abyssal lines of cognitive exclusion have historically segregated common sense and other knowledges to be suppressed of possible coupling with the hegemonic.

3.3 The Water-Energy-Food Urban Nexus and an Approach to Connect Local to Global

This section is based on a research project experience in which our team, mainly from the University of São Paulo, worked with a cutting-edge issue concerning sustainability through intersectoral and interdisciplinary framework, then employing participatory research approaches to deal with the conventional ruptures from global to local, concerned with a regular propensity of sectorized stewardship and non-democratic structures of governance.

Undoubtedly, the question of sustainability is positively associated with the challenges of urbanization and the respective issues of inequities in urban settlements as well as with the urban patterns of consumption and dependence on energy, water resources, food, among other resources from outside the cities, fostering implications in the global limits of provision. In the frame of the crisis of unsustainability within a dense complexity of intertwined scarcities, the assumption of the water-energy-food nexus (WEF nexus, or simply the nexus) arises since 2008 in the scope of international debates on global limits to economic development (Waughray 2011).

The WEF nexus is dedicated to apprehending the trade-offs among the chains of production and provision of water, energy, and food, actively recognizing reciprocal interdependencies and the need to overlap traditional siloed approaches and management. That mainstream procedures and understandings are not comprehensive enough to manage contradictions on interrelated scarcities and do not allow integrative alternatives to bring opportunities of synergies when such solutions can benefit several sectors reducing the trade-offs. However, besides a regional or global matter of scarcity, the WEF also must be understood in relation to the ethical point of view, in which billions of human beings need to have their contexts of vulnerability to be mitigated with the access to water, food, and energy to satisfy their daily demands (Hoff 2011; Harwood 2018). In this perspective of vulnerability, the WEF nexus approach must jointly address the reduction of social vulnerability as to equate the matter of scarcity and interdependency.

Some can think that the WEF nexus is a problem to be conceived and tackled at large scales to apprehend possible inventories and strategies to balance the trade-offs. Otherwise, the issue of the interdependency on the nexus crosses different territorial layers and can be related to our daily lives as the same as to the connection with a global concern. Actually, I suppose that there is no optimal territorial scale to tackle with the nexus, since in any analytical framing, the object of study will always behave like an open system. No analytical scale can embrace the completeness of the chains of water, energy, and food. Besides, the global level would embrace, but it would not be helpful to indicate real alternatives to involve social actors in their ranges of action.

Then, giving the relevance of this new perspective of rationality and the need for integrated action, the context of urban peripheries provides some peculiar scope and challenges: first, whether the matter of global scarcity must be seen as a matter of reducing vulnerability through social inclusion, then the communitarian scale can tell us how underprivileged people cope with these intertwined scarcities; second, it can be valuable to study what can be the possible connections between vulnerable people in urban settlements and the dynamics of the WEF nexus as a multilevel entity and an insight for sustainability; third, in regard to singular interest in common sense and ongoing organizational processes, it is worthy to study what community-based alternatives can be vectors of synergies within the nexus—hence, the assumption that communitarian practices and knowledges can fertilize plural alternatives to ecologize with other organizational levels contributing to generate synergies to the nexus.

This analytical local scale can also contribute to an urban nexus approach, and within such motivations, there is a possibility to assist in exploring complexities of the nexus that go beyond technical approaches, those that would minimize to balances among the water, energy, and food sectors. Moreover, approaching the nexus from the urban periphery can contribute to add layers of socio-political complexities in the scope of study and this is something that can really help to establish the nexus approach as a real and innovative contribution, and not only as one more buzzword to deal with sectoral and highly recognized issues (Cairns and Krzywoszynska 2016; Artioli et al. 2017).

In this section, recent research experience will be described to illustrate an initiative of studying the WEF in poor urban contexts applying a participatory approach. The research project was named "Resnexus—Resilience and vulnerability at the urban nexus of food, water, energy, and the environment" (2016–2019). It was an international collaboration in which three research teams had study site each and cooperation through basic chosen methods and analysis considering the heterogeneity of the three study cases, in this sense: a Brazilian team, from the University of São Paulo, coordinated by myself, studied the municipality of Guarulhos, São Paulo State, Brazil, with funding provided by FAPESP—São Paulo Research Foundation; a team from the UK, University of Sussex performed investigation in Sofia, Bulgaria, funded by ESRC—Economic and Social Research Council; and a Dutch team from the University of Wageningen, which studied in Kampala, Uganda, with funding provided by NWO—the Netherlands Organisation for Scientific Research. In this chapter, I will describe from the Guarulhos case perspective, because it is my domain, but also because in this Brazilian case, we extended the research team, objectives, and methods, giving space for a research-action approach.[1]

3.3.1 Contradictions on the Nexus in Urban Vulnerable Settlements

The historical global trend of urbanization can be understood as a search for social inclusion in a world of modernity and in a perspective of giving humans the maximal extent to choose and to change environments on their own needs and desires. But urban environments are full of contradictions in the sense of their basic premises. Deep inequities occur broadly distributed within many intrinsic layers of socio-environmental vulnerabilities and many times even some considerable "excellent" decision-making on urban planning unfold onto wicked problems (Rittel and Webber 1973).

[1] See www.resnexus.org.

A fundamental contradiction that characterizes the contemporary cities is imposed by the role of private property in a market context based on capital accumulation causing plenty of injustices and social exclusion. Such a frame has pushed forward the constant search for change and in the understanding of possibilities to conviviality with our creations (Harvey 2003). However, the pressures associated with urban iniquities are very challenging because of their causal interlinks with health and quality of life. For that matter, a search for improving environmental urban health demands integrated alternatives, innovative approaches, and the recognition of systemic interactions that support the scope of socio-environmental determinants. The issue of social inclusion and health promotion in urban contexts derives from the search for providing resources that can be very scarce and limited by interdependencies. Then, there is a need for finding integrated alternatives to be contemplated in terms of economic, social, and environmental/ecological concerns (Ottawa Charter 1986; Caiaffa et al. 2008; Kjellstrom et al. 2008; Marmot et al. 2008).

In this frame, urban vulnerability must be seen as a fundamental concern. Vulnerability in urban peripheries is intrinsically associated with poverty, rapid urbanization, inadequate access to services, employment, social protection, and health assistance. Also, environmental and occupational risks and criminal violence are associated in the frame of urban vulnerability, and this bunch of conditions can be exacerbated in the face of the global and environmental changes (Hogan and Marandola 2005; Romero Lankao and Qin 2011; Strengers and Maller 2012). Predominantly, rapid urbanization guided on economic development has driven corporative urbanization, in which the capital/companies encounter all of their needs to develop enterprises, while the surrounding society does not find its primary needs met. In certain circumstances prevalent in developing countries, the peripheralization process entails a substantial exile of communities keeping those vulnerable people without possibilities to be part of better conditions of access to the modernity benefits offered by cities (Maricato 2000; Santos 2005, 2009a, b; Holston 2009).

The urban nexus in this sense shows up as a challenge and a frame to considering necessary resources as their importance in determining social inclusion and health; moreover, it dictates the strict requirement to managing the interdependencies among sectors of scarcity, also considering the multilevel nature of the provision of water, energy, and food. The urban nexus in that frame is supposed to be helpful to work on reducing urban vulnerabilities as aggregating relevant concerns and measures on unsustainability. Anyhow, one essential point of this analysis is that people are continually dealing with nexus's scarcities in their daily lives, of course, not aware of our academic concerns and nomenclature (nexus), but with their codes, knowings, and social practices.

Getting back to the nature of self-organization in socio-ecological systems, social practices and own common sense knowings enable alternatives to survive and achieve the minimal requirements of well-being, and this is worthily remarkable in vulnerable urban contexts. With motivation in managing scarcity and material entities present at periphery contexts, social practices emerge, change and are reproduced having a relevant role to modify the social spaces or the places of practices.

Besides being intrinsic to local contexts and dynamics, social practices have nature of interactions and mediations across organizational levels; this can be understood from perspectives like from households to municipality (local) scale, or from local to global (Schatzki 2015).

Related to this and considering the necessary approximations between small urban scales and the WEF nexus, there are two sorts of contradictions relevant do consider: The first is that social practices besides being dynamic and creative are anchored in respective social spaces and also very pragmatic in dealing with constraints. Although they interact with or are mediated by social practices in different scales, it does not necessarily address problems and constraints or scarcities from other broader territorial scales. Social practices at the peripheral urban communities in such reasoning will be much more adjusted by local challenges and scarcities than with the perspective of dealing with global concerns, for instance. As already argued, the organizational capacity of communities belongs to a property to adaptive dynamics, but the reductionist science is blind to the self-organization that produces live autonomy. Moreover, the absolute disjuncture between the humane and natural reaches higher expression within modernization and urbanization, imposing difficulties to reflexive stances like acting locally as to save water and jointly reflecting on the global water crises or on the risks of severe droughts due to global climate change (Morin 2013). Then, local social practices in their dynamics and interactions are playing a decisive role at the urban communities, but almost randomly they can be positive or negative to concerns of other organizational levels. At the nexus' framework, it means that a local social practice can be synergetic or contradictory to the trade-offs within water, energy, and food demands and availability. It concurs that poverty and its consequences can generate environmental degradation and risks to public health, for example, having not enough water supply, people can inadequately store water causing contamination, wasting water, and facilitating breeding for mosquitos that spread diseases. On the other hand, better practices to save water can jointly reduce the intrinsic demand for energy, also having an effect on reducing trade-offs with food production, in that direction making a synergy to the urban nexus.

One example of a periphery social practice with synergic influence on the nexus is aluminum cans waste picking for recycling. Brazil presents one of the most efficient recycling rates of aluminum due to this waste picking practice, and this entails in reducing energy consumption and consequently mitigating trade-offs within the nexus. However, waste picking is not necessarily reflexive in this sense of an attitude dedicated to global concerns. This activity is much more observed for a quantitative influence of unemployment rates and low income of large amounts of people (Pereira et al. 2016).

The idea presented before, that there is no optimal scale to deal with the nexus, helps us to problematize this relation from local communities to other broader organizational scales. Following Benson et al. (2015), the nexus can be seen as different from other proposals of integration. For instance, the Integrated Water Resources Management that targets multi-sectoral convergence to be settled at river basins, being so water centered. The nexus makes necessary integrative dealing across preexisting structures of governance that operates in a mosaic of overlapping subsystems in different territorial scales. Let's consider a nexus approach on a macro metropolitan territory like in São Paulo State, Brazil, with more than 34 million habitants in 180 municipalities. In such a conurbation, the scales for water resources are associated with river basins in the surrounding territory; for electric energy, this region receives from Itaipu hydroelectric power plant, at the frontier with Paraguay; and in terms of food production and provision, a complex and diverse network transcends local to broader scales in the country and abroad (Giatti et al. 2016).

Such an understanding of the nexus reinforces to conceive that there is a severe challenge in reconnecting the local urban concerns and social practices associated with the nexus in convergence with the global scarcity of water, energy, and food.

The second contradiction concerning the nexus from the small urban scales is relative to cognitive exclusion. That is again the matter of fragmentation of different knowledge within a marginalizing structure. The hegemonic knowledge that supports decision-making as the reasonable prevailing alternative have no means or methods to recognize and to make approximations (structural coupling) with the local social practices and particular knowings. However, as stated before, the local ongoing processes of searching for alternatives in the adaptive sense make contexts that have always been ignored. Moreover, the barrier imposed by hegemonic thinking imposes the abyssal line again. For that matter, if in a periphery community, people develop innovative and synergetic practices within the nexus, it probably will not be realized as something to build hybrid knowledge and problem-solving in association with governmental planning and action.

In summary, there is a rupture challenging for more sustainable and healthier contexts: it is characterized by the two contradictions that make marginalized the local social practices with potential to deal with the nexus and engender more sophisticated, diverse, inclusive, and fair alternatives. These contradictions are related to the need for reconnecting cross-territorial concerns and to the lack of knowledge democracy. So, for those who live in an urban periphery like in Guarulhos, their practices and knowings must be encompassed in the process of legitimate inclusion on the issue of sustainability. This inclusion must be social and cognitive, and it must pave a cross-sectoral pathway of dialogical interactions, connecting them with the global issue of scarcity, passing through the conditioning related with the constraints in the macro metropolitan region in which Guarulhos is implicated.

This kind of related rupture is what I have called nexus of exclusion (Giatti et al. 2019). On the assumption of interdependencies among water, energy, and food, this concept is related to the impossibility of vulnerable people to have conscious decisions as well as to take reflexive behaviors connecting their daily life attitudes to broader scales of interaction with sustainability and also the lack of perspective to merge their knowings and practices with the hegemonic rationality and decision-making.

3.3.2 Methods for Apprehending the Nexus and Searching for Synergies in Urban Communities

The presentation of methods and results here is an attempt to describe proceedings to approach the nexus making this concept attainable to the context of an urban peripheral and vulnerable community. There is an intent to bringing alternatives to approximate local contexts, knowings, and practices to the two kinds of contradictions introduced above. So, much more relevant than empirical results and the methodological steps are the processes and approximations, in this sense showing possibilities for collaborative learning and problem-solving, building a dialogical interaction among local residents, practitioners, decision-makers, and researchers. Above all, the first challenging task was to understand how the nexus can be implied in the daily lives of vulnerable urban people.

The qualitative methods applied to apprehend the nexus in the peripheral urban community was an ethnographic approach associated with participatory workshops as the main agenda of investigation of the ResNexus project, during 2017 and 2018. Besides this, two other subprojects were carried out: a Participatory Geographic Information System—PGIS approach; and an urban garden participatory implementation.[2]

The site of the study was the community of Novo Recreio, a peripheral neighborhood in Northern Guarulhos municipality (1,200,000 inhabitants), which is in a conurbation with São Paulo municipality, the biggest city in Brazil (more than 11 million inhabitants). Novo Recreio has approximately 4500 households and has limits to the Cantareira State Park, a permanent preservation area. The community has had low and intermittent water security, lack of sewage collection, and besides receiving a regular collection of household waste, several sites show trash accumulation. The neighborhood has a landscape of plateaus and slopes characterizing risks of erosion and landslides (see Fig. 3.1).

The shadowing ethnographic approach had focus on investigating each person at a time as to describe particular social practices of interest in the study, in this case, mediations pertinent to the access and use of water, energy, and food, as well as possible interconnections (McDonald and Simpson 2014). The theoretical background was the Theory of Practice (Nicolini 2012; Schatzki 2015), exploring: (1) how specific actions have been constituted over time; (2) how others may emerge or disappear, and (3) how they can evolve and relate to other actions. It retains the assumption that these actions are in ongoing development and change, and continuously subject

[2]As the research involved human beings through qualitative research, it was in line with international standards of ethical criteria, such as free and informed consent, voluntary participation and the possibility of withdrawing at any time, and assurance of confidentiality of information provided and identity of participants. Young participants up to 18 years old had informed consent signed by responsible guardians. Although there was a diversity of collective activities as in the community meetings, in which the local social actors interacted among them and with researchers, the confidentiality was assured in terms of analysis, discussion, and dissemination of the research outcomes.

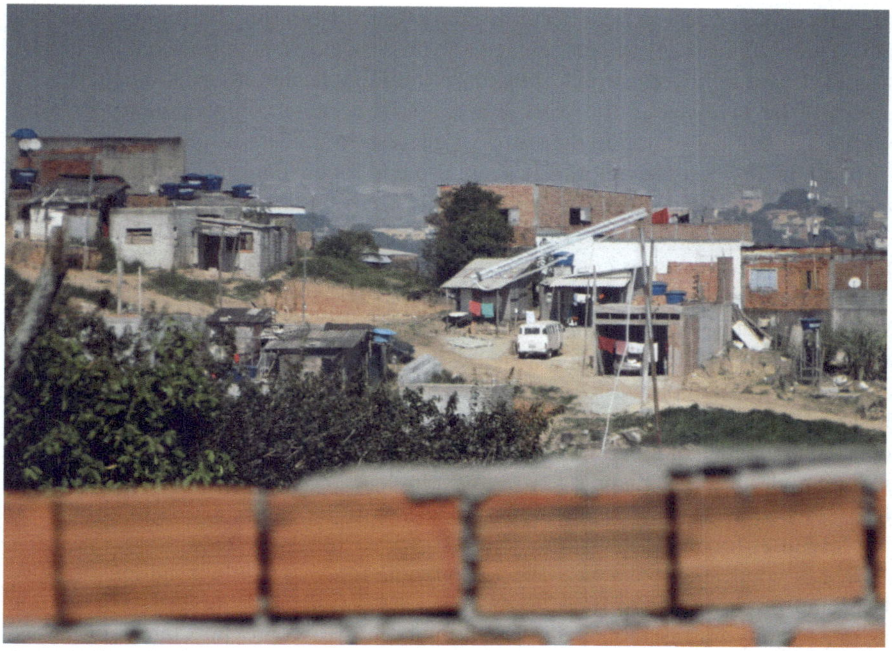

Fig. 3.1 Novo Recreio neighborhood in Guarulhos, 2018. (Source: the author)

to negotiation and contestation. These actions are social practices that are co-created with knowledges and then being "places" for knowing. In other words, knowledge manifests itself within and through a practice (Nicolini 2011, 2012; Schatzki 2015).

Fieldwork was carried out through visits to 12 households in Novo Recreio, direct observation of local dynamics and collection of secondary data from public institutions. The public primary health care professionals facilitated the activities at the neighborhood, it was mainly necessary to make successful visits to households for attending to the criteria of exploring qualitative narratives and diversity of situations associated with the nexus. Additionally, conversations with health professionals, teachers, and professionals of the local Municipal School and visits and conversations with small local commerce helped to generate empirical data (Giatti et al. 2019).

Besides the ethnographic fieldwork, the participatory approach was held at three workshops involving residents, primary health care team, and professionals from the public school of Novo Recreio. Other participants of the workshops were from outside the community: researchers from the University of São Paulo; and professionals and decision-makers from some municipal secretariats like environment, health, and social services. In the workshops, there was an application of participatory research tools like the river of life (Wallerstein et al. 2017) and world café (Fouché and Light 2011). The third workshop, carried out as a world café, also had the attendance of researchers from the international team (the University of Sussex and University of Wageningen). Hence, the process of research involved the collection of data at fieldwork, which subsidized finding relevant information, and social actors to be involved in the workshops, which became complementary to work within a dialogical stance on the issues of interest. More details related to processes of participatory research approaches and use and sequencing of participatory tools are presented in Chaps. 4 and 5.

The first subproject associated was on the PGIS approach carried out in 2017 through a 30 h extension course offered to 22 young students (14–17 years old).[3] The course was offered in a local NGO by the University of São Paulo, which provided certificates to the participants. It was a process of applying successive research tools like "talking maps," "photo panels," and "community newspaper", promoting reflection and collaborative learning (Toledo and Giatti 2014) on socio-environmental local concerns. The development of interactions made possible the gradual introduction to the idea of the nexus, its components (water, energy, and food), as well as several trade-offs. The mapping process explored the context in which young people live (see Fig. 3.2), also considering their lack of resources like access to leisure and opportunities for social inclusion.

The second subproject was the implementation of an urban garden in Novo Recreio from late 2017 to June 2018 when there was the first harvesting. It became an opportunity for research and intervention because of a previous interest between two relevant local institutions: The Primary Health Care Unit and the local Municipal School, this last provided the site for implementing the garden. Having such a previous interest, the researchers identified a real possibility for collaborative work on building alternatives aligned to synergy towards the nexus. An urban garden can be understood as something to optimize the resources of the nexus, reducing trade-offs, but also involving people to produce food and simultaneously managing and reflecting on energy and water limitations. Following the methodological design of participatory research action (Thiollent 2011), this subproject joined efforts from local residents, health care, and school professionals to work together from the planning for implementation, acting, reflecting, and bringing their personal agricultural skills and knowledge to make possible the realization of the garden. The respective process also involved participatory research tools and a significative amount of collective work (Honda 2018).

3.3.3 People and the Nexus: Insights for Reconnecting

The amount of empirical data provided by the different work fronts in research brought a sort of relevant narrative. Besides this, the characteristic of interaction and collaborative learning made possible dialogical progress on the issue of the nexus

---

[3] This initiative is related to the post-doctoral project of Carolina Monteiro de Carvalho on my supervision, funded by FAPESP (proc.n. 2015/21311–0), and held in the School of Public Health of the University of São Paulo.

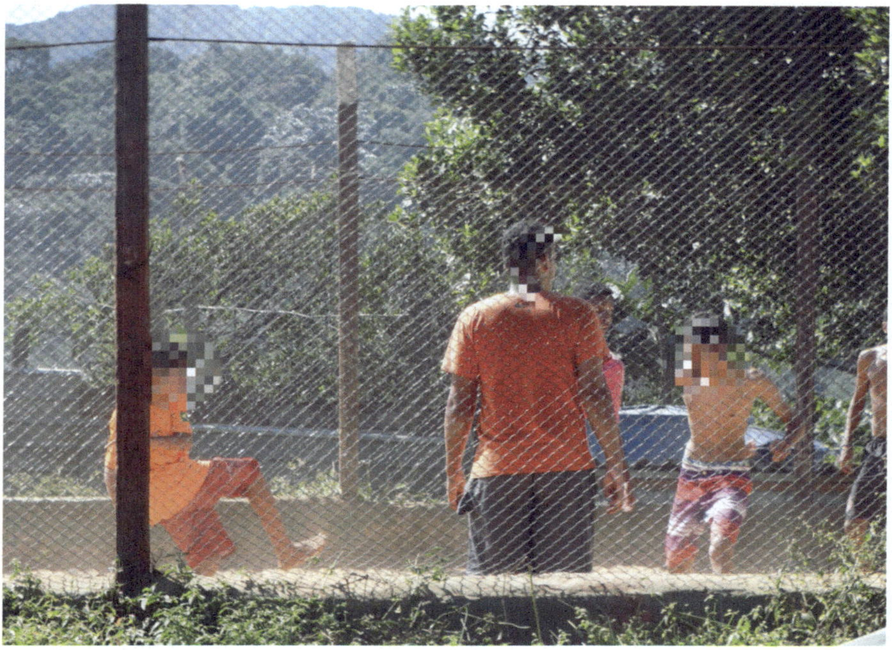

Fig. 3.2 Young people playing soccer in Novo Recreio—at the back the protected areas of natural rainforest, which limits the neighborhood. (Source: the author)

and respective connections with communitarian daily life, professional activities of health agents and school workers, and also some positive approximations with decision-makers from the municipality occurred.

At first, it is possible to emphasize the relevance and the nature of data generated by the ethnographic investigation. In this segment of the research, narratives were analyzed about social practices contextualized spatially and temporally in the urban periphery, as so concerning elements of the nexus. Thus, the social practices were classified as related to how people mobilize water, energy, and food chains and scarcities creating specific arrangements of contradictions or synergies within the nexus. In other words, characteristics of the studied practices were classified as their potential to aggravate or to relive the burden of the trade-offs of the intertwined scarcities, then providing a picture on aspects of vulnerability mitigation. The social practices studied showed association with relational knowledge—knowings and doings—mediated by material constraints and artifacts, and rooted in an interaction context (Nicolini 2011).

Besides the scenario of lack of public investments, sanitation, and other urban infrastructures, the investigation also demonstrated other prominent attributes of the studied spaces of practices in Novo Recreio. Thus, a general economic context of poverty was observed, insecurity of not having land titles—part of the neighborhood is settled informally or in protected natural areas. Moreover, other constraints were lack of sanitation with the risk of contamination of local water resources that are regularly withdrawn for some residents, hilly topography worsening urban transportation, and geographical isolation that makes difficult transportation to have access to jobs, higher literacy, and public services like secondary level health care.

Water scarcity is a central concern in nexus thinking (Hoff 2011), and in Novo Recreio, as in the whole Guarulhos city, the intermittent public water supply challenges vulnerability reduction and connects the study site with other territorial scales, like that of the macro metropolitan context of hydrological risk and territorial interdependencies (Jacobi et al. 2015). Accordingly, the nexus approach can make possible reasonable approximations with the daily practices of dealing with the scarcity and the intrinsic multilevel circumstances.

To cope with the intermittency of water supply, residents store water in plastic barrels or other containers. For those with higher income, water tanks are installed on the roof of dwellings. The precarious water storage creates other vulnerabilities like the possibility of contaminating water or breeding for mosquitos that can transmit diseases like dengue fever or yellow fever. When some dwellers are without water supply, sometimes they withdraw water from a local spring, seriously threatened by contamination due to the absence of sewage collection and treatment. The occasional local withdraw of water is also hindered by the hilly topography.

Surprisingly, there is an incongruity in the low perception of the lack of water since it has not appeared as one of the local most important problems for the studied families. It is argued that the social practices assume an important role by means of perceiving the space and possibilities, even though with the surrounding context that presents contradictions within incapacity to attain a fair quality of life, negative health-related issues, and being in a region that suffers the worse consequences of the broader territorial problem of water scarcity. Such a setting discloses a background of resignation in the face of the oblivion and the lack of public policies and social inclusion initiatives. Otherwise, it makes sense to understand that the social practices and associated knowledge—the connection of knowings and doings—(Nicolini 2011) must play a relevant role to promote social and cognitive inclusion, dealing with sustainability and public health.

Concerning energy, the verified topics were transportation, electric energy access in households, and public street lighting. Due to the geographical isolation, the prevalent transport modal is by public buses that are scarce, taking too long to reach other parts of Guarulhos city, like downtown, and being intermittent in hard rainy days because of lack of pavement of streets that give access to Novo Recreio. Some streets do not have public lighting, and a response sometimes is given by residents, providing street lighting on their own, then replacing lack of public investments. In terms of access, some households receive electrical connection at subsidized rates, and some steal energy through clandestine connections; both alternatives make imbalance and possible indiscriminate consumption or wasting of energy. A very positive aspect related to energy is the local prominence and regular activity of collecting recyclable materials to sell, strengthening the chain of recovery energy in parallel with complementing family income.

Acquisition of food was registered as a very central element in the context of the nexus in the community. Similarly to other urban peripheries, the central conditioning for that was the low availability of fresh and healthy food, and the tendency to prevail the offer of processed or ultra-processed food that corroborates with population malnutrition status. Thus, those peripheries have been understood as food deserts (Cummins and Macintyre 2002; Lang and Rayner 2002; Hendrickson et al. 2006; Ver Ploeg 2010; Duran 2013). According to Santos (2009b), the low income of residents discourages local trade and services. When local trade exists it is constrained by a shortage of supplies and relatively high prices. It corroborates to difficult access to the local provision of fruits and vegetables and facilitates selling industrialized food. Then, to acquire fresh food, it is necessary to go out of the neighborhood, which contrasts with the question of the geographic isolation interplaying a trade-off with the energy necessary for urban transportation.

In this analysis, exploring the nexus as a practical set of measures for sustainability in Novo Recreio, food can be placed in a central analysis, also having great relevance for the contemporary context of public health; once poor people of urban peripheries like in Brazil are becoming obese in fast transition. Analyzing the nexus centered on the food acquisition issue in Novo Recreio makes to consider that for reducing vulnerability and promoting social inclusion, it is necessary to find alternatives for providing fresh and healthier food locally. Production and transportation of food demand water and energy, in this sense, producing food locally can reduce the trade-offs, representing alternatives for sustainability in association with the idea of food sovereignty (Azevedo 2015).

There is a family who farms vegetables in Novo Recreio, and it was observed as a remarkable synergy with the nexus. In the community, they grow and sell lettuce, parsley, chives, cabbage, coriander, clove lemon, and manioc. Such social practices contribute to local sustainability as it fills a fundamental gap, providing fresh food. To fertilize the garden, they use manure, partly produced locally, and for irrigation, preferably they use rainwater. It is relevant to stress this sense of joined and cross-sectional perspective of nexus-friendly alternatives, with the power to deal with issues conventionally isolated by silos. Such interactions bring simultaneous benefits like reducing the trade-offs among water, energy, and food chains, involving local people in relevant solutions, and fostering health promotion (Ottawa Charter 1986; Kickbusch 2003). That is a substantive acknowledgment of sophistication: a local social practice with multiple entanglements across sectors and also converging with the far-reaching intents of the Sustainable Development Goals (UN General Assembly 2015; Buss et al. 2016). As stated before, the diversity of doings and knowings in a community, through the ongoing creation of alternatives, is anchored in the local space of practices, but these practices can be very pertinent to positive interactions with problems in other scales, like those concerning the global crisis of unsustainability. Anyhow, the disconnection due to the cognitive exclusion seems to be still present, the farmers are not necessarily growing food in consideration of the need for a global sustainability goal, and the local public power conveniently ignores the local farmers' activities as well as their role in local food production, sustainability, and health promotion. So, that is a background to reinforce the concept of nexus of exclusion.

On the power of local food production concerning the nexus and health promotion, the initiative of implementing an urban community garden was considered as an excellent opportunity also for dialogical interactions through participatory action research. Moreover, as there was prior interest on behalf of some local residents and health and school professionals, the coincidence made a good start for this participatory action enterprise, also giving an opportunity to encompass the issue of the nexus at local community social actors. It is worthily a good beginning because a previous wish converted in initial social mobilization is something essential to begin the participatory research. Sometimes researchers went to communities imbued with highly relevant problems like some related to health determinants, but if the chosen issue is not of urgent interest to the community, the process of starting necessary collaborative activities can be laborious.

Still, on the process of social mobilization feasibility, the nexus thinking was very far from the local cultural background, and its premises would not be comfortable to facilitate interaction among researchers and local social actors. Thus, the implementation of the urban garden, as compatible with a previous local desire, was the opportunity to delineate a pathway to connect these two worlds that are so different. The academic assumption of the nexus aligned to a discourse of sustainability and public health could encounter the communitarian "codes" that connect the subjects with the objective and concrete reality, represented by food, agricultural skills, a sense of belonging to the community, work, land, seeds, among other materials. The challenge in having successful participation in this sense was to promote a journey of ongoing departures and comings from the abstract—the academic assumption of the nexus—to the concrete, the social spaces of practices in local context.

The collaborative work involved 19 people from the community, primary health care, and municipal school. The meetings were held biweekly interplaying participatory research tools but much more dedicated to collective work. The process was cyclical in which the analysis of empiric data from each activity provided feedback for planning or redesigning further actions. Stakeholders, involved as subjects, were engaged in making collective decisions and planning as well as to finding solutions for the shortfall of resources, like supplies to cultivate, and addressing the need to build flowerbeds, as indicated for cropping in the site provided by the municipal school. Subjects organized a local bazaar to obtain money, invited a volunteer bricklayer to build flowerbeds (see Fig. 3.3), and asked for local commerce donations of materials, like cement. The dialogical interactions made possible that the knowledge applied to the garden implementation was the one constituted of subjects' previous agricultural knowledge (Fig. 3.4), enabling a process of constant and collaborative teaching and learning, concomitantly of a collection of doings.

To analyze the participatory implementation of the garden, a Community-based Participatory Research (CBPR) framework was applied to the process, helping to evaluate the results (Hicks et al. 2012; Oetzel et al. 2018). Table 3.1 shows the synthesis which can be understood in a logical sequence through four interactive dimensions of a socio-ecologic model. In such a framework, the dimension of con-

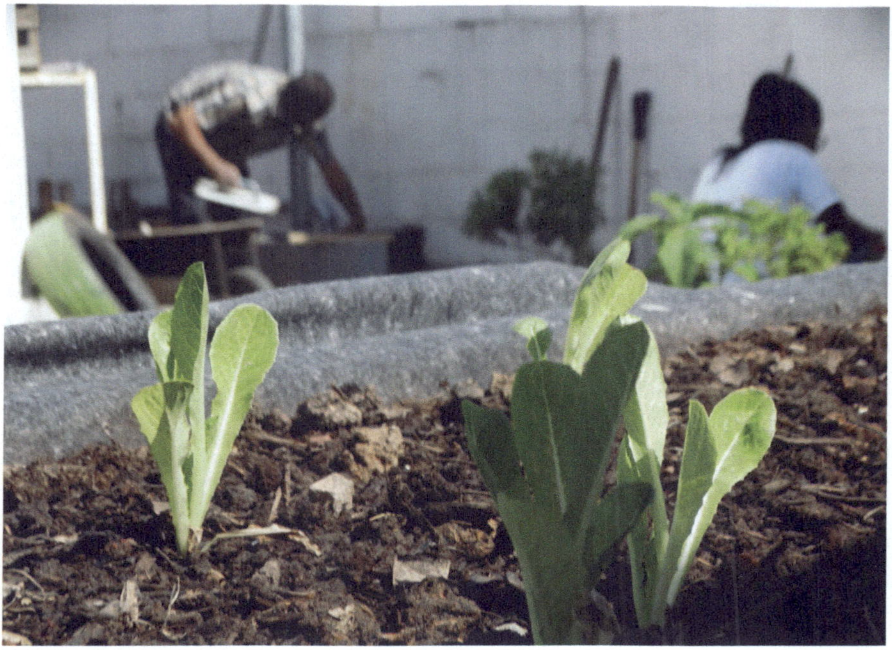

Fig. 3.3 Local partnership for action—the volunteer bricklayer building flowerbeds. (Source: the author)

text is elementary for any participatory trial, but the dimension of partnership processes appears as something significant and with the property of optimizing scarce resources through the strengthening or establishment of partnerships. A singular opportunity for a partnership was the municipal program named "Ambienta Saúde,"[4] which targeted supporting environmental health actions to be held for primary health care units. Thus, such a program provided know-how and resources for implementing the garden, for instance, roof tiles to build flowerbeds and amount of organic compound to crop. The dimension of intervention and research points out the main strategies and actions, responsible for the core of the participatory and dialogical process. Finally, the CBPR framework showed the dimension of outcomes, some being intermediate in association with the process and some long term as contributions to the community that relates to empowerment, self-esteem, and social capital.

The first harvest was in June 2018 with the attendance of the social actors involved, young students from the school, local partners, and researchers. This event was very

[4] "Ambienta Saúde" is an intersectoral program of the Guarulhos municipality launched in 2017 and headed by the Health Secretariat; its objectives are associated with searching improvements on socio-environmental local issues, like waste management, water and sanitation, energy consumption, urban forestation, biodiversity, responsible consumption, and zoonosis control.

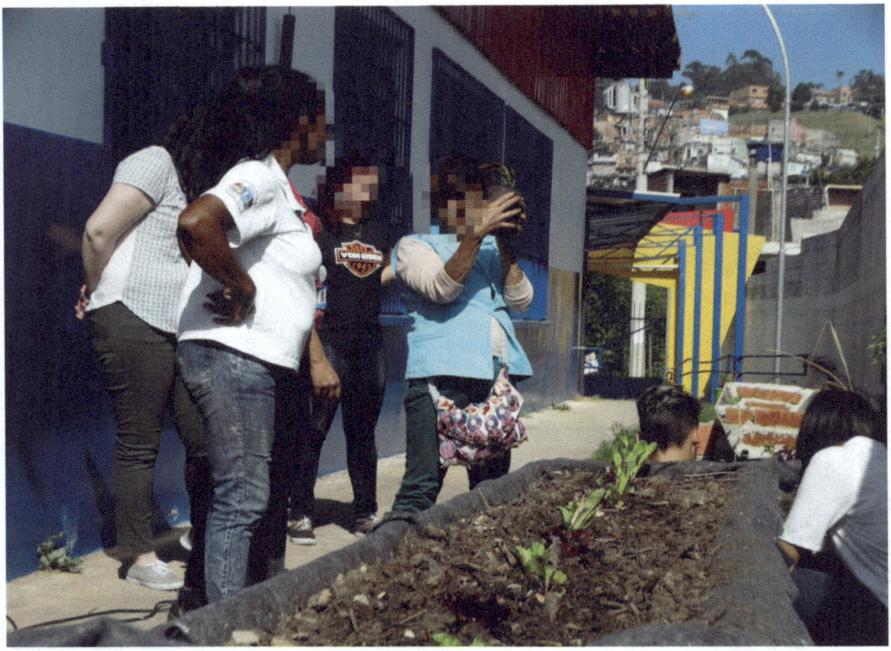

Fig. 3.4 Exchanging agricultural knowings and doings in Novo Recreio, Guarulhos, 2018. (Source: the author)

Table 3.1 CBPR framework applied to the implementation of an urban garden in Novo Recreio, Guarulhos, Brazil, 2018

Contexts	Partnership processes	Intervention and research	Outcomes
– Socio-environmental vulnerability – A previous desire to have an urban garden – Available space at the school – Difficult access to resources – Agricultural knowledge among people from the community	– Primary health care, municipal school, and university cooperation – "Ambienta Saúde" municipal program/policy – Local people cooperation – Local commerce donations – Volunteer bricklayer	– Workshops and collaborative work at the urban garden (cyclical approach), participatory research tools, meetings – Beneficent bazaar with donations – Flowerbeds, cropping, irrigating, harvesting	Intermediate: – Successful first harvesting – Involvement of community – Contribution for educational measures Long term: – Empowerment – Self-esteem – Social capital

Elaborated by the author with data adapted from Honda (2018) relevant as to prove to the local stakeholders that it is possible to perform results from collaborative projects in contexts of scarcity and lack of resources and opportunities. Moreover, it made feasible the desired interaction among nexus assumptions and the search for alternatives from the community, as a bottom-up process.

The PGIS activities were an opportunity to work with young people putting them in the discussion on local urban planning as to think about local attributes inherent to socio-environmental context and also to do an exercise on conceiving alternatives to deal with the lack of public investments and perspectives for social inclusion and better quality of life. Geographic Information Systems—GIS are very straight as used on the domain of academics and decision-makers with technical support. Since then, traditionally, the ways of practicing urban planning with such technical respect make the characteristic division of lines in which common sense and regular citizen are out of the processes, then GIS can be a part of the frontier delimitating such different worlds. The exercise of PGIS was the opposite and can be considered a prominent innovation to approximate people from an urban periphery to the language and the technological tools as well as to the rationality of critically reflecting on their own space, problems, possible choices, and rights. Young people from peripheries demonstrated themselves as very distrusting of the researchers and the proposals of the PGIS at the beginning, but the continuing process of participatory research could make for better interactions.

A PGIS process can be a very fruitful and democratic initiative, for instance, in consideration that frequent participation in master plans is something considered as a right with a legal guarantee, but there is no formal application of proper instruments to make such participation tangible and winning. For that matter, PGIS constitutes an integrative tool that on the one hand can gather relevant data from a broad range of citizens, and on the other hand, can help people to make necessary reflections and to be aware of their rights, their power, and their possibility to assume a participative stance. This kind of integration also reinforces more transparency in procedures and decisions and fosters commitment among decision makers and citizens (Kahila-Tani et al. 2016).

The bundle of initiatives in Novo Recreio generated a set of ethnographic evidence. At the same time participatory methods such as workshops, PGIS course, and the implementation of the community garden added supplementary narratives. In other words, it made possible a system of interactions throughout a process of investigation and participatory activities, making it possible that all the social actors could learn in the ongoing interactions. So, the team of researchers from the University of São Paulo has learned much more than acquiring data from the application of traditional research tools, like interviews or other local non-participatory data collection. The academics could learn in cooperation with young people and with people dedicated to the implementation of the community garden. More about these systemic interactions and the gains in terms of learning will be detailed in Chap. 4. Anyhow, it is foremost to recognize that researchers had to work together with residents to find all the local alternatives, attainable partnerships, and agricultural knowledge to make successful the garden.

Local residents could learn by their interaction and also by interacting with the themes, ideas, and challenges brought by the researchers. Health professionals, workers, and teachers from the local school also learned even about their strengths and the possibility to work in collaboration with the university and with the local residents. Decision-makers likewise, although they were not always involved, being requested and present in a few meetings, could play an essential role in the interaction in the final workshop of the ResNexus project. This workshop was in June 2018, also having the presence of foreign researchers.

That was a significant moment for all the social actors to get involved in a dialogical activity. For residents, for instance, only the previous and continuing participatory processes could get them engaged enough to have voice and prominence in this final workshop. For researchers, the dialogical stance could help in knowing better the residents and then having pathways to build reciprocity and symmetrical environment necessary to reach the objectives of collaborative and balanced interactions involving social actors from such different insertions. As the language of the workshop was Portuguese, foreign researchers had constant assistance from translators (Portuguese–English) at expository moments and during the collaborative discussions of the world café. This final workshop could merge these processes of collaborative learning and research and with this provide some narratives of the building of hybrid knowledge. Some narratives are presented below, as they helped deepening the understanding of the local context.

Water unavailability appeared to affect health professional's performance in the reality of the general scarcity at the neighborhood, also in terms of health care. One day, the doctor of the Primary Health Care Unity had 100 medical appointments, then the water came to Novo Recreio, and only 50 people attended to the booking. When having to manage the intermittent water supply, sometimes when the water comes, it is necessary to dedicate priority for managing such a scarce resource, having additional work on storage, or being obligated to wash accumulated clothes.

Also related to the intermittent water supply, people argued that the Guarulhos' water company was a hostage of SABESP—a mixed economy company controlled by the state government of São Paulo, that used to sell water to Guarulhos. That is a perception of people from Guarulhos that shows a reflexive point of view on the matter of water scarcity through different scales and the interplay of institutions and levels of governance. This range of vision shared by people from Novo Recreio, professionals, researchers, and decision-makers shows the possibility of having a connection among the daily life social practices associated with the lack of water and the multi-layered problem or water resources.

Regarding the completeness of the nexus issue, some participants stated that solutions must come not only from the authorities (decision makers) but also from the communities and citizens. Of course, it was not something to justify the lack of public policies aiming the periphery. Instead, it was the recognition that the community could be relevant to create appropriate solutions and the decision-makers should be aware of this perspective of the binding interaction.

Regarding energy issues, because of the high elevation price of bottled gas from 2016 to 2017, it was found that some people were opting for the microwave for cooking. This concerned only people with subisidezed access to electric energy or those who steal energy. That is a relevant point to be investigated as a topic of efficient use of energy. Anyhow, it also showed that there was a conflict, a social tension between those who pay for electric energy and those who pay less or do not pay for such source of energy.

The activity of waste-picking for recyclables was also reported, but with a judgment that in the face of lack of training, those waste-pickers sometimes become accumulators of materials, and it can bring secondary problems to environment and health.

Reinforcing acquisition of fresh food, participants discussed the relevance of strengthening local knowledge to cope with the distorted information that comes from media, which often provides a wrong idea associating industrialized food as a symbol of social status. Such an assumption also called attention for the need for more understanding and planning on food systems and associated aspects of production and food distribution, as something to play a relevant role in sustainable development and health. Some previous actions also came to a new understanding concerning the neighborhood, for example, the local school had promoted a few activities on producing sustainable and healthier alternatives, and it encouraged the proposition of more prominence for the school that could organize communitarian kitchen to learn and teach how to cook without wasting. This alternative marked an integrative view and action concerning the nexus, as well being friendly to food security.

Related to the successful participatory process of the community garden implementation, a decisive statement came from a communitarian health agent that participated: She said that when the project of the garden started there was no belief in the possibility of achievement, but eventually, after her and others' work and involvement, it became a concrete reality, overlapping a myriad of small bottlenecks and constraints. The assertion showed two fundamental aspects at the spectrum of challenges of participatory research involving vulnerable people: first, in the beginning, the lack of trust and low self-esteem; second, the realization of empowerment, making it possible that with local resources, knowledge, and partnerships, people from the community can achieve common objectives.

The final workshop of this research also had the objective of joint reflection on possible futures with alternatives that could address more or less sustainable scenarios in consideration of the nexus. The researchers being the facilitators of interaction among social actors pursuing relevant targets, the team worked on driving the discussions on the perspective of mitigating the nexus of exclusion, which would be to decrease the vulnerability in association with regard to finding choices to approximate people from the community with understandings, constraints, and actions on other scales. So, that was an attempt to dedicate effort in opposition of the classically stipulated ruptures.

Many topics appeared together in the sense of working on reducing the nexus of exclusion and the vulnerability in the urban periphery. The issue of urban sustainability, for instance, is a primal and contemporary challenge that must consider the dependence of urban systems from other territorial dynamics. Cities are the core of human activities connecting global spread networks of production, demand, and consumption. Besides, it is in cities that many innovative options can make difference in mitigating process that threaten planetary boundaries like climate change due to greenhouse gas emissions (Ernstson et al. 2010).

The supposition of a nexus as a more sophisticated rationality can also occupy a relevant status in managing alternatives and connecting sectors and scales conventionally disperse or isolated. In this sense, the target of reducing trade-offs among sectors with previous governance structures and siloed management distinguishes the beginning of this proposition of nexus thinking in my assumption. In fact, another fundamental matter in that direction is to establish or (re)connect the global lack and intertwined scarcities with the contexts of local constraints and social practices. The urban peripheries, where a massive number of inhabitants live together with poor access to water, energy, and food, present the most sensitive issue on rupture, that is, the situation in which social practices are forged continuously to manage local constraints, but being prone to engender contradictions or synergies. Building bridges on such a rupture is something to operate with doings and knowings, linking local dynamics and understandings with other scales and public policies.

Approaching the nexus must be through multilevel and multi-stakeholder platforms that enable participatory and bottom-up arrangements. It does not necessarily mean at creating new mechanisms, but encouraging relations of actors from multiple domains, like business and finance, knowledge production, and citizens. The interaction and respective actors' issues must contribute to understanding a nexus governance and searching for alternatives through the lens of the nexus thinking (Boas et al. 2016; Howarth and Monasterolo 2017).

The ResNexus project in Novo Recreio, Guarulhos, was not enough to manage all of these aspects converting lasting solutions. However, it built means for interaction and reflection, bringing together social actors that traditionally are very distant, sometimes maintained apart by power, hierarchical relations, and cognitive exclusion. In this process steered by participatory research, it was also possible to accomplish a nexus-friendly alternative, the community garden that besides the small but significative production of food could propitiate learning at distinct levels, also inducing relevant problem-solving and pushing forward a local empowerment process.

With this transversality in public policies involving dialog with community people and across sectors emerged something achievable and necessary to search for urban resilience and vulnerability reduction. Moreover, the nexus-friendly alternatives and focal issues like fresh food acquisition or local food production were highlighted and made a sense in the co-creation of new knowledge in searching for integrative solutions. This form of new knowledge is not only created in collaboration of different social actors but indeed they share it. The forms of appropriation of this collaborative knowledge will be conditioned by the differences in context of the social actors involved. That is a process to establish trust and reciprocity among social actors divided by hard historical relationships. Moreover, it must be seen as necessary to deal with the complex and multilayered issues of sustainability, health, and vulnerability reduction.

3.4 Reflexive and Liberation in the Freirean Philosophy Applied to the Current Contexts

A significative element on sustainability debate is scarcity, associated with interdependencies with subordination to the need to access and to manage common-pool resources like irrigation systems, forest resources, inshore fisheries, groundwater basins, and intrinsic chains of dependence (Ostrom 2009). The fundamental assumption on this critical issue is pointed out by Hardin in his classic paper "the tragedy of the commons," in which technological pathways were evidenced as controversial to the matter of scarcity when applied on commons, then being necessary to recognize moral concerns on systemic limits and relativize the need to access resources (Hardin 1968).

With more integrated and contemporary understandings on socio-ecological systems, Ostrom (2009) makes significative contribution characterizing institutional diversity and the role of sophisticated structures of multilevel governance bringing workarounds to such elementary issues related to sustainability. Besides the high level of complexity, some common dilemmas have demonstrated interrelated self-organizing responses to cope with the tendency of collapse. However, there is a need to understand such complexity as to improve the perspectives of sustainability, and this challenge concerns to recognizing operational rules on different organizational levels, the role of social actors and institutions, cultural backgrounds, and the nature and protagonists in action arenas—those which are related to the process of dealing with the resources limitations and disputes concerning demands. Action arenas are the place of decision and conflicts of interests on the scarcities, and such arenas can be interrelated through different levels of organization in a holarchic frame. For instance, a communitarian constraint treated within a local attitude represents a set in whole (holon), but at the same time this territorial cutting belongs to and is interdependent of the same kind of scarcity dynamic in a broader level, also as another whole (or system), like a city, or a river basin, successively (Kay et al. 1999).

For enhancing the efficiency of such interdependent multilevel structures, there is a need to search for better interactions among different levels and across the nested organizations present at any level. Transparency and accountability, as well as social inclusion, are relevant to permeate and to improve justice and the quality of these necessary interactions, delivering better outcomes in the sense of preventing systemic failures with collapses in the dimensions of resources (ecological), society, or economy.

However, power and asymmetrical relationships can prevail in the scenarios of scarce resources like the entanglements of the global water crisis, in conjunction with conflicts and imbalanced excluding structures of water management that can be referred to as "hydrocracies." Such frameworks involve complex administrative components characterizing policy making operated mainly on water sector conceptions, frequently guided by the power of technical groups, like civil engineers, dictating relevant strategies like decisions to open new catchments, negotiation with publics, priorities for water supply, and a general trend on choosing for substantial construction of alternatives with high levels of investments. The prevalent technical rationality, as can be verified in United States, Peru, Bolivia, Mexico, and in Brazil, can be negligent to the existence of deep inequalities in water supply and environmental constraints or risks of deep scarcities. Also, such technical domain is often related to institutional history in a context of entrepreneurially competing for power and financial recourses, and it supports controversy as to boosting water supply instead of considering how the resource is used or limited (Poupeau et al. 2018).

The research on water governance as cited in the Americas shows the burden of highly concentrated power supported by the hegemonic domain of technical and scientific knowledge, converging to rationality that not only excludes social actors in vulnerable conditions but also keeps those marginalized people far from the mainstream decision and action arenas. If in Ostrom's assumptions there is a consistent recognition of possible self-organizing and interrelated search for mitigating risks of chaos, the conventional power structures substantiate decision-making in the track of maintaining the cognitive exclusion and related inequities. Furthermore, such stances can operate in overshadowing vested interests behind positivistic affirmatives and decisions.

Whether more sophisticated structures of multilevel governance are possible and required for sustainable development goals, then it is necessary to understand and to act on reducing the differences and the process of dispossession of rights and access to resources that is kept through marginalization of minorities, which occurs in parallel with the denial of vulnerable peoples' knowledges and representativeness.

Moreover, one additional aspect in this problematic is that uncertainties clearly permeate the current dimension and nature of risks, otherwise, as in the related case of water resources management, the technical rationality continues to keep uncertainties away in the name of promises of lasting solutions that rely on the positivist basis of problem-solving (Ravetz 2004). Like other situations of our late modernity, there is dispossession of necessary reflexive interactions, and it retains inertia, simplification of knowledge, and unpreparedness on emergent risks.

The recent critical experiences with the most severe water crisis suffered in the Metropolitan Region of São Paulo, Brazil, can illustrate and provide some lessons on these conventional structures of power, related decision-making, and unjust adverse consequences (Buckeridge and Ribeiro 2018). Between 2013 and 2015, a sequence of unprecedented droughts made to hit the lowest level of water in the reservoirs available for this metropolis of more than 20 million inhabitants. It was the hardest drought period verified since the previous 80 years of registering rainfall index. The possible association of this drought with the global phenomena of climate change stayed below the scientific evidence until now, but it was understood as a remarkable anomaly as an intense disturbance on the natural climatic variability. Anyhow, this critical incident showed the vulnerability not only of the metropolitan but of the macro metropolitan system in the state of São Paulo, with more than 34 million inhabitants.

A central component of the crisis was the Cantareira system of water supply that was implemented in the 1980s as a "lasting" solution, bringing water since the state of Minas Gerais, and disputing water resources that naturally flowed to the region of the Campinas metropolitan region, the second biggest conurbation in the interdependent macro metropolitan territory. At the crisis, such a system used to supply water for eight million inhabitants, mainly in São Paulo capital city, in a network with a lack of alternative distribution because of the absence of hydraulic connections with other systems of supply. Cantareira system, whose related river basins are in regions of less rainfall incidence, became almost waterless, inducing a constraint of millions of people without any other option for water supply. Besides that, the dispute of water due to the implementation of Cantareira exacerbated the very dramatic lack of options for the Campinas region, where there is no dam for water reservation until now.

The overconfidence in the conventional decision-making based on major infrastructure of water brought from distant places, with lack of options for integration, denoted incapacity to have preparedness for a severe crisis—little safety margins to cope with uncertainties. This frame made evident the high hydrological risk and the way that such a scope has always ignored local water resources and alternatives of reuse of water, keeping wastewater treatment rates low, and insufficient investments in reducing high distribution losses and unaware consumption.

Implications of the crisis came in the form of disputes, risks of systemic failures, rationing of water supply mainly for the most distant and poor neighborhoods, and lack of transparency and accountability, primarily related to ignoring the seriousness of the crisis and the selective water shortage. The relationship among uncertainties, values in dispute, high stakes (even electoral issues), and the need for urgent actions characterized an unquestionable post-normal problem. Yet, the management of these issues was strictly "normal", since technical assumptions prevailed and uncertainties were ignored. Besides the characterization, within this normal problem-solving and concentration of power, the whole society was not empowered in order to critically control the process of decision-making based on technical solutions.

Social movements raised and organized themselves in forums denoting the imminent social struggle, strongly related to the iniquities, like people in poor urban peripheries suffering contingency of water supply. Anyhow, such a scenario, corroborated by unfair water shortage, drove the recognition that neither previously nor during the crisis there was any possibility for protagonism on behalf of those vulnerable people in the conventional structure of governing water resources in the State of São Paulo. That was the extensive fracture in the perspective of democratic, interactive, and necessarily multilevel structure for water governance. In this case, it was obvious the circumstance in which people of the community could deal with their local practices on given conditionings, not reaching the determinants of the vulnerable context and power arenas. Such iniquities in water supply exacerbated by a very severe drought showed the disruption circumstantially maintained by social and cognitive exclusion. Also, such a scenario was corroborated by a previous lack of dialogical reflections on the uncertainties and hydrological risk.

The condition of having the power to decisively interact on action arenas for more democratic governance of resources can be seen as a matter of liberation from such oppressive and centralized structures. The rigid and conventional structures seem to suppress the autonomy of social actors that is naturally diverse. In other words, that is a framework that represses self-organizing properties, mainly from the level of the community. It relates to an anti-dialogical action.

In addition, this mainstream centralized structure can also hinder a sort of different structural couplings of alternatives and distinguishable demands that could result in more diverse, integrated, wise, fair, and resilient systems. Ruptures and impediments in that sense also affect the ability of mutual and necessary learning. Thus, people from vulnerable communities do not find adequate translations to become aware and in proactive stance. On the other side, the status quo does not allow or have means to understand the possible role of a plural society as a requirement for the sustainability of such systems. For that matter, knowledge gaps are on both sides, of the dominant and of the excluded. This context relates to what Freire (2000) called the theory of oppressed action, shown in Fig. 3.5, which reproduces itself in an anti-dialogical unilateral relationship from actors–subjects (dominant elites) to oppressed people, placed as objects.

Coping with the anti-dialogical conventional structure related to a complex and uncertainty permeated issue requires sophisticated and permanent reflexive interactions, empowerment, and democratic postures. In that direction, Paulo Freire's (2000) theory of revolutionary action provides some relevant elements to encourage dialogical practices to involve social actors. Promoting humanization and intersubjectivity among subjects–actors in the ongoing pedagogic process, this is a long-standing framework that is helpful to overlap the abyssal distance among different knowledges and understandings. In effect, previous well-succeeded practical experiences supported Freire through adult literacy and in that way, the culture circles was a crucial fieldwork tool that assisted with the methodological development (Freire 2018).

The approach for the theory of revolutionary action consists of a dialogical cultural action, considering that liberation from oppression must be born from social entities, through legitimate participation. Circles of culture can be useful for this, but also other kinds of participatory tools can be applied (see Chap. 4). The

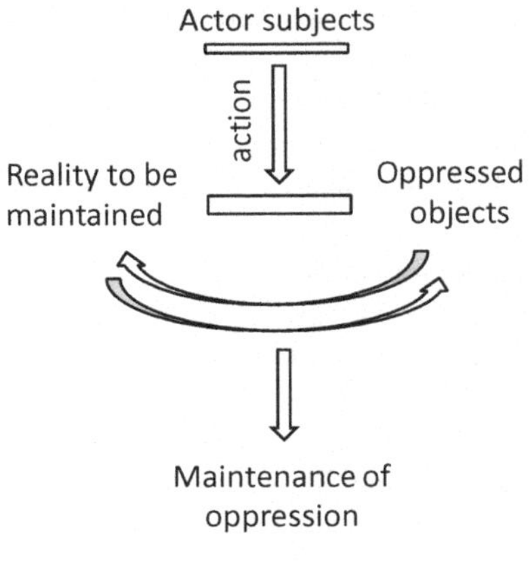

Fig. 3.5 Theory of oppressive action. (Source: adapted from drafts of Paulo Freire (1968 in Silva 2017))

researcher–educator must work as a mediator for guiding the activities to stimulate interactions among subjects. At the beginning of the dialogical interaction, the subjects will be brought into the dynamic of identifying generative themes, those with local relevance at their life and work, as critical forms of thinking and acting about their world. Investigation of generative themes means at instigating subjects to think about their reality and their need and alternatives to act upon such a reality, understanding and finding ways to change contradictions.

Generative themes can be conceived as concentric intertwined circles, and their problematization can come throughout units and subunits, as coming from global to local and multilayered issues. So, in the context of the ruptures in our societies, considering the relation of hegemonic knowledge and decision-making and the peripheric condition of cognitive exclusion, generative themes at any level must be related to subjects' perception of their world in their scale of regular interaction. Within the small/local circles where subjects can be implied, like in the context of a small community, they must have the possibility to navigate from their concrete reality to the abstract world of other temporal and time scales.

As the subjects in their cultural contexts develop their own ways to apprehend the reality, then a successive process of coding and decoding situations in analysis must operate to move from the concrete to the abstract, making possible translations and interactions among social actors from different cultural backgrounds (like researchers and people from a vulnerable community). Such a process also means as the interplay between being a subject and recognizing himself or herself as an object of interaction. In that way, "subject recognize himself in the object (the coded concrete existential situation) and recognize the object as a situation in which he finds himself, together with other subjects" (decoded) (Freire 2000, p. 105). The evolving moves make it possible to cease barriers of impenetrable realities, as also fostering reflection, reciprocity, and possibilities of action. That is a liberation process once the subjects realize themselves from concrete reality to others before unreachable total realities.

Paulo Freire (2000) in *Pedagogy of the Oppressed* considered as a primary aim to address domination, and so liberation as a necessary response. Today, we have to target issues with the characteristic of post-normal problems, like climate change, related uncertainties, and the possibility of a myriad of consequences on different socio-environmental vulnerabilities. We also have to engage the theory of revolutionary action with the issues of multiple and sometimes antagonistic stakes, controversies and values, unprecedented emergent impacts, and the need to find prompt alternatives to unknown systemic consequences. Anyhow, the contemporary problems of uncertainties and the complex issues of unsustainability and health-related issues are also holders of differentiated oppression relations and also domination.

Figure 3.6 is a proposal to encompass a representation of the theory of revolutionary action on the background of complexities and uncertainties associated with contemporary post-normal problems. In the middle vertical axis, there is the process of dialogical interactions boosting intersubjectivity that is the axis and the direction of an evolving process (see Chap. 4). On both sides, we see axes representing social actors, to the left, the subjects–actors with the commitment of changing realities through symmetrical and collaborative stance. That is the reason why those actors can be understood either as teachers or researchers in the Freirean assumptions. As researchers, they join in the process also with the perspective of transforming themselves and changing the reality in a political protagonism (Brydon-Miller et al. 2003). On the other side, to the right, the vulnerable people, recognized as oppressed, are represented as subjects, in recognition of their possibility and demand for being a part in the process of change. This figure illustrates from the perspective of a libertarian education, based on dialogical interaction involving primarily teachers and students. However, as demonstrated, it can be applied to involve other social actors, as in community-based participatory research, for instance, should engage together researchers and local dwellers implied in socio-environmental vulnerability.

Moreover, the same rationale could be applicable for involving other social actors in multilevel approaches (see Chap. 5), constituting other lateral axes to promote an extended system of interactions. For example, in a context of urban water supply scarcity and iniquities, a multilevel approach could proceed to engage urban periphery residents, researchers, policy-makers from the municipality, and representatives and institutions committed with water governance in the level of a river basin in which the target municipality is enclosed. That is a proposal to extend the dialogical interactions to cope with the multilayered complexities, promoting reflections on uncertainties, and obligatorily fostering better and fairer structures of

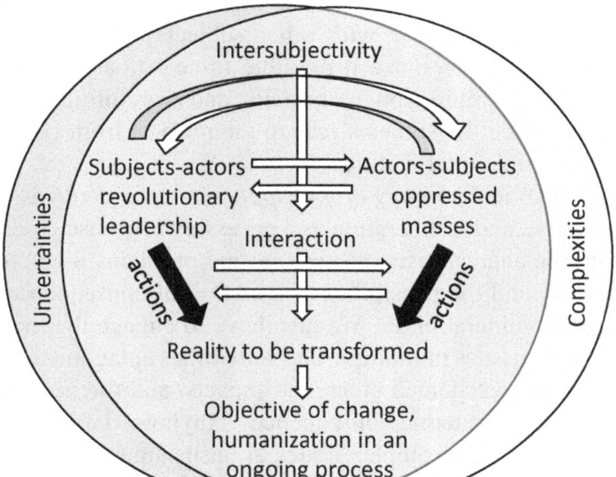

Fig. 3.6 Theory of revolutionary action in the background of uncertainties and complexity. Source: adapted from drafts of Paulo Freire (1968 in Silva 2017). (Both Fig. 3.5 and this figure were adapted from unpublished Paulo Freire's handmade drafts. Originally those drafts were conceived for the book *Pedagogy of the Oppressed* in 1968, when the author was living in exile in Chile, where the drafts remained in possession of friends until 2000, when the figures and other material were donated to Instituto Paulo Freire in Brazil (Silva 2017)

governance with partnerships and convergent actions of social actors in different organizational or territorial levels.

Comparing the distinguishable nature of interactions between Figs. 3.5 and 3.6, the last represents in essence the need for participatory processes to face the complex contemporary issues permeated by uncertainties, requiring deep, ongoing, and multi-stakeholder reflections and social learning. In an applicable way on the cutting-edge issue of the WEF nexus, Stirling stresses the radical need to "broaden out" and "open up" (Stirling 2015, p. 25) about nexus-related methodologies. Such a proposal considers the implication of distinct social actors, knowledges, and institutions, interplaying objectivity and subjectivity of necessary stakeholders in the process. In that way, framing the understanding on nexus and the possibilities of dealing with such uncertain matrices of causes and consequences requires a range of different capabilities, possible linkages, and interventions, taking into account policy interventions to engage with a greater diversity of alternatives and ways of understanding. Once the ruptures of social groups and institutions through cognitive exclusion is mainstream, the dialogical action on promoting bridges for social actors' interactions seem to be a primary attitude to deal with complex issues of unsustainability and health-related consequences.

References

Artioli, F., Acuto, M., & Mcarthur, J. (2017). The water-energy-food nexus: An integration agenda and implications for urban governance. *Political Geography, 61*, 215–223.

Azevedo, E. D. (2015). O Ativismo Alimentar na perspectiva do Locavorismo. *Ambiente & Sociedade, 18*, 81–98.

Bauman, Z. (1999). *Modernidade e ambivalência*. Rio de Janeiro: Zahar.

Bawden, R., Guijt, I., & Woodhill, J. (2007). The critical role of civil society in fostering societal learning for a sustainable world. In A. E. J. Wals (Ed.), *Social learning towards a sustainable world: Principles, perspectives, and praxis* (pp. 133–147). Wageningen: Wageningen Academic Publisher.

Benson, D., Gain, A. K., & Rouillard, J. J. (2015). Water governance in a comparative perspective: From IWRM to a 'nexus' approach? *Water Alternatives, 8*, 756–773.

Boas, I., Biermann, F., & Kanie, N. (2016). Cross-sectoral strategies in global sustainability governance: Towards a nexus approach. *International Environmental Agreements: Politics, Law and Economics, 16*, 449–464.

Brydon-Miller, M., Greenwood, D., & Maguire, P. (2003). *Why action research?* Thousand Oaks: Sage Publications.

Buckeridge, M., & Ribeiro, W. C. (2018). Livro branco da água. In *A crise hídrica na Região Metropolitana de São Paulo em 2013-2015: Origens, impactos e soluções*. Instituto de Estudos Avançados.

Buss, P. M., Fonseca, L. E., Galvão, L. A. C., et al. (2016). Health in all policies in the partnership for sustainable development. *Revista Panamericana de Salud Publica, 40*, 186–191.

Caiaffa, W. T., Ferreira, F. R., Ferreira, A. D., et al. (2008). Saúde urbana: "a cidade é uma estranha senhora, que hoje sorri e amanhã te devora". *Ciência & Saúde Coletiva, 13*, 1785–1796.

Cairns, R., & Krzywoszynska, A. (2016). Anatomy of a buzzword: The emergence of 'the water-energy-food nexus' in UK natural resource debates. *Environmental Science & Policy, 64*, 164–170.

Christopher, S., Watts, V., McCormick, A. K. H. G., & Young, S. (2008). Building and maintaining trust in a community-based participatory research partnership. *American Journal of Public Health, 98*, 1398.

Cummins, S., & Macintyre, S. (2002). "Food deserts"—Evidence and assumption in health policy making. *BMJ: British Medical Journal, 325*, 436.

da FL Duuran, A. C. (2013). *Ambiente alimentar urbano em São Paulo, Brasil: Avaliação, desigualdades e associação com consumo alimentar*. São Paulo: Universidade de São Paulo.

Díaz, S., Pascual, U., Stenseke, M., et al. (2018). Assessing nature's contributions to people. *Science 359*:270–272.

Ernstson, H., Van der Leeuw, S. E., Redman, C. L., et al. (2010). Urban transitions: On urban resilience and human-dominated ecosystems. *Ambio, 39*, 531–545.

Fouché, C., & Light, G. (2011). An invitation to dialogue: 'The world café' in social work research. *Qualitative Social Work, 10*, 28–48.

Freire, P. (1985). Reading the world and reading the word: An interview with Paulo Freire. *Language Arts, 62*, 15–21.

Freire, P. (2000). *Pedagogy of the oppressed* (M. B. Ramos, Trans.); *Introduction* (D. Macedo, Trans.) (30th anniversary ed.) New York City: The Continuum International Publishing Group Inc.

Freire, A. M. A. (2018). *Paulo Freire: uma história de vida*. Editora Paz e Terra.

Gell-Mann, M. (1995). *The quark and the jaguar: Adventures in the simple and the complex*. London: Macmillan.

Giatti, L. L., Jacobi, P. R., Favaro, A. K. M., et al. (2016). O nexo água, energia e alimentos no contexto da Metrópole Paulista. *Estudos Avançados, 30*, 43–61.

Giatti, L. L., Urbinatti, A. M., & Carvalho, C. M, et al. (2019). *Nexus of exclusion and challenges for sustainability and health in an urban periphery in Brazil*. Cadernos de saude publica 35:e00007918.

Hall, B. L., & Tandon, R. (2017). Decolonization of knowledge, epistemicide, participatory research and higher education. *Research for All, 1*, 6–19.

Harari, Y. N. (2016). *Sapiens: uma breve história da humanidade. 12. Traduçao: Janaina Marcoantonio*. Porto Alegre: L&PM.

Hardin, G. (1968). The tragedy of the commons. *Science, 162*, 1243–1248.

Harvey, D. (2003). The right to the city. *International Journal of Urban and Regional Research, 27*, 939–941.

Harwood, S. A. (2018). In search of a (WEF) nexus approach. *Environmental Science & Policy, 83*, 79–85.

Hendrickson, D., Smith, C., & Eikenberry, N. (2006). Fruit and vegetable access in four low-income food deserts communities in Minnesota. *Agriculture and Human Values, 23*, 371–383.

Hicks, S., Duran, B., Wallerstein, N., et al. (2012). Evaluating community-based participatory research to improve community-partnered science and community health. *Progress in Community Health Partnerships: Research, Education, and Action, 6*, 289.

Hildebrand, M., & Bunyard, P. (1993). Gaia and culture: Reciprocity and exchange in the Colombian Amazon. In *Gaia in action* (pp. 248–265). Edinburgh: Floris Books.

Hoff, H. (2011). *Understanding the Nexus: Background Paper for the Bonn2011 Nexus Conference*. SEI.

Hogan, D. J., & Marandola, E. (2005). Towards an interdisciplinary conceptualisation of vulnerability. *Population, Space and Place, 11*, 455–471.

Holston, J. (2009). Insurgent citizenship in an era of global urban peripheries. *City & Society, 21*, 245–267.

Honda, S. L. O. (2018). *Pesquisa-ação na implantação de horta comunitária: empoderamento e sustentabilidade na periferia de Guarulhos*. Master Thesis, Faculdade de Saúde Pública—Universidade de São Paulo, Brasil.

Howarth, C., & Monasterolo, I. (2017). Opportunities for knowledge co-production across the energy-food-water nexus: Making interdisciplinary approaches work for better climate decision making. *Environmental Science & Policy, 75*, 103–110.

Jacobi, P. R., Cibim, J., & Leão, R. v. S. (2015). Crise hídrica na Macrometrópole Paulista e respostas da sociedade civil. *Estudos avançados, 29*, 27–42.

Kahila-Tani, M., Broberg, A., Kyttä, M., & Tyger, T. (2016). Let the citizens map—Public participation GIS as a planning support system in the Helsinki master plan process. *Planning Practice & Research, 31*, 195–214.

Kay, J. J., Regier, H. A., Boyle, M., & Francis, G. (1999). An ecosystem approach for sustainability: Addressing the challenge of complexity. *Futures, 31*, 721–742.

Kickbusch, I. (2003). The contribution of the World Health Organization to a new public health and health promotion. *American Journal of Public Health, 93*, 383–388.

Kjellstrom, T., Friel, S., Mercado, S., et al. (2008). *Our cities our health our future. Acting on social determinants for health equity in urban settings*. Report to the WHO Commission on Social Determinants of Health from the Knowledge Network on Urban Settings.

Kropotkin, P. (2012). *Mutual aid: A factor of evolution*. North Chelmsford: Courier Corporation.

Lang, T., & Rayner, G. (2002). *Why health is the key to the future of food and farming: A report on the future of farming and food*. Centre for Food Policy, Thames Valley University: London.

Lazenbatt, A., Lynch, U., & O'Neill, E. (2001). Revealing the hidden 'troubles' in Northern Ireland: The role of participatory rapid appraisal. *Health Education Research, 16*, 567–578.

Lucero, J. E., Wright, K. E., & Reese, A. (2017). Trust development in CBPR partnerships. In N. Wallerstein, B. Duran, J. G. Oetzel, & M. Minkler (Eds.), *Community-based participatory research for health: Advancing social and health equity* (p. 61). San Francisco: Jossey-Bass.

Magnani, J. G. C. (2002). De perto e de dentro: notas para uma etnografia urbana. *Revista Brasileira de Ciências Sociais, 17*(49), 11–29.

Maricato, E. (2000). Urbanismo na periferia do mundo globalizado: metrópoles brasileiras. *São Paulo em perspectiva, 14*, 21–33.

Marmot, M., Friel, S., Bell, R., et al. (2008). Closing the gap in a generation: Health equity through action on the social determinants of health. *The Lancet, 372*, 1661–1669.

Maturana, H. R., & Varela, F. J. (1992). *The tree of knowledge* (rev. ed.). Boston: Shambala.

McDonald, S., & Simpson, B. (2014). Shadowing research in organizations: The methodological debates. *Qualitative Research in Organizations and Management, 9*, 3–20.

Moran, E. F. (1991). Human adaptive strategies in Amazonian blackwater ecosystems. *American Anthropologist, 93*, 361–382.

Morin, E. (2013). *A via para o futuro da humanidade*. Rio de Janeiro: Bertrand Brasil.

Nicolini, D. (2011). Practice as the site of knowing: Insights from the field of telemedicine. *Organization Science, 22*, 602–620.

Nicolini, D. (2012). *Practice theory, work, and organization: An introduction*. Oxford: Oxford University Press.

Oetzel, J. G., Wallerstein, N., Duran, B., et al. (2018). Impact of participatory health research: A test of the community-based participatory research conceptual model. *BioMed Research International, 2018*, 7281405.

Ostrom, E. (2009). *Understanding institutional diversity*. Princeton: Princeton University Press.

Ottawa Charter. (1986). *Ottawa charter for health promotion*. First international Conference on Health Promotion, 17–21 November 1986, Ottawa, Canada. Retrieved June 26, 2019, from https://www.who.int/healthpromotion/conferences/previous/ottawa/en/

Pereira, T. N. D., Milanez, B., Moreira Filho, R. M., & de Almeida Nogueira, F. M. (2016). *A Reciclagem De Alumínio No Brasil E O Mercado Internacional: Uma Análise Quantitativa*. Planejamento e Políticas Públicas.

Peterson, G., Harmáčková, Z., Meacham, M., et al. (2018). Welcoming different perspectives in IPBES:"Nature's contributions to people" and "Ecosystem services.". *Ecology and Society, 23*, 39.

Poupeau, F., Razafimahefa, L., & Robert, J, et al. (2018). *Water conflicts hydrocracy in the Americas: Coalitions, networks, policies*. IEE-USP.

Raine, K. D., Plotnikoff, R., Nykiforuk, C., et al. (2010). Reflections on community-based population health intervention and evaluation for obesity and chronic disease prevention: The healthy Alberta communities project. *International Journal of Public Health, 55*, 679–686.

Rand, D. G., & Nowak, M. A. (2013). Human cooperation. *Trends in Cognitive Sciences, 17*, 413–425.
Ravetz, J. (2004). The post-normal science of precaution. *Futures, 36*, 347–357.
Rittel, H. W., & Webber, M. M. (1973). 2.3 planning problems are wicked. *Polity, 4*, 155–169.
Rockström, J., Steffen, W., Noone, K., et al. (2009). A safe operating space for humanity. *Nature, 461*, 472.
Romero Lankao, P., & Qin, H. (2011). Conceptualizing urban vulnerability to global climate and environmental change. *Current Opinion in Environmental Sustainability, 3*, 142–149. https://doi.org/10.1016/j.cosust.2010.12.016.
Santos, M. (2005). *A urbanização brasileira*. Edusp.
Santos, B. de S. (2009a). Una epistemología del sur: la reinvención del conocimiento y la emancipación social. Siglo XXI
Santos, B. d. S. (2007). Para além do pensamento abissal: das linhas globais a uma ecologia de saberes. *Novos estudos-CEBRAP, 79*, 71–94.
Santos, M. (2009b). Metrópole corporativa fragmentada: o caso de São Paulo. In *Coleção Milton Santos*. Editora Edusp.
Santos, B de S., Araújo, S., & Baumgarten, M. (2016). As Epistemologias do Sul num mundo fora do mapa. In *Sociologias* (pp. 14–23). Universidade Federal do Rio Grande do Sul.
Schatzki, T. (2015). Spaces of practices and of large social phenomena. *Espaces Temps 24*.
Silva, C. T. da. (2017). *A gênese da Pedagogia do Oprimido: o manuscrito*. PhD Thesis, Universidade de São Paulo.
Snyder, T. (2017). *Sobre a tirania: Vinte lições do século XX para o presente*. Editora Companhia das Letras.
Steffen, W., Broadgate, W., Deutsch, L., et al. (2015). The trajectory of the Anthropocene: The great acceleration. *The Anthropocene Review, 2*, 81–98.
Stirling, A. (2015). *Developing 'Nexus capabilities': Towards transdisciplinary methodologies*.
Strand, R. (2017). Post-normal science. In *Routledge handbook of ecological economics* (pp. 288–298). London: Routledge.
Strengers, Y., & Maller, C. (2012). Materialising energy and water resources in everyday practices: Insights for securing supply systems. *Global Environmental Change, 22*, 754–763.
Thiollent, M. (2011). *Metodologia da Pesquisa-Ação* (18th ed.). São Paulo: Cortez.
Toledo, R. F., & Giatti, L. L. (2014). Challenges to participation in action research. *Health Promotion International, 30*, 162–173.
UN General Assembly. (2015). *Transforming our world: The 2030 Agenda for sustainable development, A/RES/70/1*. Retrieved June 27, 2019, from https://sustainabledevelopment.un.org/content/documents/21252030%20Agenda%20for%20Sustainable%20Development%20web.pdf.
Ver Ploeg, M. (2010). *Access to affordable and nutritious food: Measuring and understanding food deserts and their consequences: Report to congress*. Collingdale: Diane Publishing.
Von Bertalanffy, L. (1968). General system theory. *New York, 41973*, 40.
Walker, B., Holling, C. S., Carpenter, S. R., & Kinzig, A. (2004). Resilience, adaptability and transformability in social–ecological systems. *Ecology and Society, 9*, 5.
Wallerstein, N., Duran, B., Minkler, M., & Oetzel, J. G. (2017). *Community-based participatory research for health: Advancing social and health equity*. Hoboken: Wiley.
Waughray, D. (Ed.). (2011). *Water security the water-food-energy-climate nexus: The world economic forum water initiative*. Washington, DC: Island Press.
Wolowski, M., Agostini, K., Rech, A. R., et al. (2018). *Relatório Temático sobre Polinização, Polinizadores e Produção de Alimentos no Brasil*. Brasil: BPBES.

Chapter 4
Adaptive Methods

4.1 Self-Organization in Participatory Research

Participatory research approaches must be seen as systems of interaction, keeping in mind ongoing processes of fostering dialogical relationships among researchers and subjects[1] through collaborative learning in a process that can have different objectives, but always must contribute toward balanced interactions in consideration of classically asymmetrical correlations. Participatory approaches must work on necessary approximations, not only as an imperative for cognitive justice but as a need to reconnect different worlds that have suffered varied fragmentations, like the conventional concentration of power and knowledge steering social exclusion, or the vast distances separating vulnerable people from complex and emergent risks due to the side effects of modernity.

Reconnecting such distant knowledge systems must be understood as necessary to attain the challenging and multifaceted contemporary problems. In that way, participatory processes are choices that can promote approximation and interaction of a myriad of knowledges and social practices, making possible structural couplings through different social actors and several organizational levels. It means at overlapping the disconnections that were established by the division in hegemonic and marginalized knowledges, which have caused a rupture in the natural property of self-organization—concerning autopoiesis, which enables self-transformation in the process of creating alternatives, interacting and changing the surrounding reality (Maturana and Varela 1992).

[1] Following Freire in *Pedagogy of the Oppressed* (Freire 2000), the term "subject" represents those who know and act, and it is in contrast to an "object," where once in the banking concept of education educators deliver knowledge to students. The freirian pedagogy is applied here conceiving the relationships among researchers and subjects, because the proposal is a process of collaborative learning, then, both actors research and learn at the same time. And the subjects are recognized for the emancipatory view in which they can transform their world, and doing so toward new possibilities of richer life experiences, individually and collectively.

L. L. Giatti, *Participatory Research in the Post-Normal Age*,
https://doi.org/10.1007/978-3-030-27924-0_4

Particularly on the post-normal problems, participatory approaches must perform a fundamental role, bringing a broad range of stakeholders to critically control the relationship among science and decision-making. It can create opportunities for those that suffer huge impacts of complex consequences and uncertainties, enabling voice and possibility to decide, mainly when there is no scientific certainty on questions of high stakes, with the possibility of severe and systemic impacts.

The expectations on these concerns are very high, note that some conditioning of the mentioned ruptures has been established and reproduced over centuries. So, the results are not so fast and straightforward to attain. Actually, there must be a diversity of possible applications for participatory approaches, varying in terms of the extent of the process of interactions, or pursuing different objectives, like making a collaborative diagnosis, local problem-solving, or empowering people to have legitimate prominence and voice in more democratic structures of governance. Anyhow, what is very important to remark is that a participatory project must be carried out as a system of interactions that depends on true involvement of researchers and subjects and also must be cyclical and adaptive (List 2006; Toledo and Giatti 2014; Baum 2016). That is foundational, and for that matter, researchers must be entirely aware of their role to facilitating necessary approximations and symmetrical relationships, also keeping the disposition to constant reflections and adaptive methods, considering insights, desires, interests, and decisions on behalf of the subjects.

Projects and initiatives carried out within participatory frameworks are associated initially with the democratization of knowledge; otherwise, very frequently, such endeavors must cope with problems with determinants intrinsic to structures of power and exclusion, relationships and consequences of globalization and colonialism, and contexts of huge and tacit inequities. The acquisition of outcomes in a participatory approach in that way must request much assertiveness, commitment, and interactions in the medium or long term. In the sense of reaching democracy as a continuous pursuit, participatory approaches must be encouraged as essential for successful and legitimate representation on issues of common interest. In other words, a continuous process of social struggle to repair ongoing forces that tend to capitalize themselves on the developments and maintenance of cognitive exclusion.

On behalf of researching targets in a participatory approach, initially, I would like to mention the character of generating narratives and reflections as singular qualitative results related to the process of interaction among different social actors and the associated collaborative knowledge produced. Otherwise, the strategy of combining different research tools, as also some classical research instruments, in association with the subject's participation can result not only in objective and quantitative answer, but also in trust and reciprocity, mutual learning, and empowerment. However, considering the process of participation as a system of interactions, it is quite relevant to stress that replication is not achievable in a relation of the uniqueness of a multifactorial conditioning, reflections, and qualitative narratives produced. Such systems of interactions must be realized as singular processes of producing knowledge, a kind of new knowledge that will be relativized for the scope of intersubjectivity, anchoring the reflexive results to the view of the social actors involved, in a specific moment of their personal histories, with current scenarios, power relations, needs, and desires. That is a process continuously humanized carried out through actions, and it really must be like this to attain the quality and reciprocity in participation.

The concept of post-normal problems seems to require new societal models to absorb and reflect on scientific production as well as to induce more dynamic, fast, and self-organizing possibilities of relations among science, society, and decision-making. Indeed, as uncertainty, rapid change, realignment of power, and chaotic behaviors characterize our age, there is a clear recognition of more compelling, adaptive ways of knowledge production. The required transition is absolutely on virtues of humility, modesty, accountability, and the indispensable recognition of living with uncertainty, complexity, and levels of ignorance (Sardar 2010). It relates to accepting new and adaptive production of knowledge through participatory processes with a level of unpredictability in the intersubjective interactions, rethinking on the classical perspective of replicability and the dogmatic and conventional normal science, which cannot be continuously applied in solving the complex contemporary issues.

The rupture with the dogma of replicability opens a window for stepping across the abyssal rupture between science and common sense. It represents an exchange that begins with the academic disposition of sharing power and then representing a stance to understand that in legitimate participatory processes, the researchers do not have to take full control of the research. In that way, a remarkable issue in my concern is to assimilate better this nature of driving an intervention without the perspective that the results must be replicable. However, on the other side, the exchange comes making it possible to receive true collaboration, to build trust through reciprocity among researchers and subjects.

All of this process is entirely related to power; hence, the lines that divide science and common sense are determinants of structures in which those who have the domain on science also have more possibility to decide or to conduct private entrepreneurship, projects, or dispossessions. In this sense, the decision on conducting participatory research is a political decision and represents a disposition to giving up power for empowering those people that are classically viewed as objects of research, turning them into subjects.

4.2 Cyclical and Adaptive Methods

The issue of establishing legitimate and dialogical involvement is what requires ongoing processes as a system of interactions, but it also can be responsible for continued production of actions, outcomes, decisions, and social and cognitive inclusion. So, how can it be the onset of a participatory project? It depends on a variety of factors, for example: how much is the concern and the motivations for a participatory project prioritized among the subjects? It can be a real and relevant problem, but maybe the stakeholders can be engaged in other problems of more urgency, or even their perception does not match the issue argued by the researchers. The related experience of Iauaretê (Chap. 2), with the indigenous population in the Brazilian Amazon, on sanitary conditions shows that it was not a priority for them, although those people used to have significant mobilization on fighting for primary health care (Toledo et al. 2012).

Otherwise, sometimes the issue is a recognized demand presented by the subjects, even having social capital aggregated, but lack of instrumental assets to deal with the problem, like the case of the indigenous people in Ecuador, in the struggle on the environmental and health consequences due the oil industry impacts (San Sebastián and Hurtig 2005).

Both at the beginning and during the whole participatory process, social mobilization on the related problem is quite fundamental, as well as trust building and maintaining. Also, and not less relevant, there is a need for constant dialogical interaction, employing adequate language and connecting people with their visions of the world. This connection with common sense can be possible, for example, with the proposal of exploring generative themes, and the interplay among the concrete reality of the subjects and the subjective understandings (Freire 2000), which can be related to the academic knowledge as to be exposed and interpreted by the subjects.

Social mobilization towards the problem is focal for participation and can be understood as the first challenge to fostering a system of interactions. When a group of people, community, or society has the stance for acting based on a common objective or problem, then it characterizes social mobilization. Otherwise, the lack of such collective will can also be expressed within some kinds of resistance to research, an inertia of the population and low perception on common issues, and also the prevalence of low self-esteem (List 2006; Toledo and Giatti 2014). Lack of social mobilization as an initial constraint to participation seems to be more significant when the studied problem is not presented initially as a self-determination from the subjects (Cargo and Mercer 2008), as exposed in the case of indigenous of Iauaretê in Amazon, which was concerned with health care but not with the issue of water and sanitation.

After having started the process, and keeping in mind the importance of continually nurturing social mobilization, the participatory research can have its own "life" through the development of collaborative work and application of participatory tools. The system of interactions can be understood with the properties of self-organization through cyclical dynamics, aggregating various social actors (with their knowledge, expectations, desires, perceptions, and experiences), making possible their perspective of autonomy, and the possibility to interact in searching for collaborative knowledge, collective solutions, and cognitive inclusion. With this, both subjects and the system of interaction (the participatory process) possess the property of autopoiesis, which is to promote change when interacting with a problem/circumstance, at the same time transforming themselves in the process (Maturana and Varela 1992).

Cyclical dynamics in participatory research have been proposed and applied by Lewin (1946) in the 1940s, contributing to minorities' engagement in a series of subsequent planning, acting, and fact-finding. Since then, and to the current times, some contributions have been applied and collaborated to the application and coverage of such cyclical and ongoing procedures. For instance, in CBPR, the premise of involving the subjects in all the phases of the research shows similarities in the sense of ongoing and reflexive participation within a continuum of community engagement (Wallerstein et al. 2017a, b). The proposal of adaptive and integrative governance on risks also makes a relevant contribution to highlight the need for stakeholders' participation in a cyclic and continuous process of dealing with uncertainties and complexities through collaborative work on pre-estimation of risks, monitoring and controlling, interdisciplinary estimation, characterization, evaluation, and management (Klinke and Renn 2012).

List (2006) also makes a relevant systematization of continuous phases on the progress of participatory approaches, identifying through practical experience the level of commitment and social mobilization, also indicating the search for the highest level to be pursued, which is of the proactive stance and empowerment. The expectation is that at first there are communities with low self-esteem, disperse social capital, and low mobilization to manage their collective problems, and the participatory research can gradually contribute to changing the scenario of lack of power, inaction, and disperse capacity of responses.

In the same direction, Toledo and Giatti (2014) also presents a continuing process to deal with challenges to participate in action research, ordered as follows:

1. Social mobilization, as the start or a previous stance of the subjects to act on a common problem
2. Cooperation, through the successful application of participatory tools bringing identification of the subjects with the research, making them more prominent in the process and fostering dialogical participation
3. Appropriation, addressing cognitive re-signification of knowledge through intersubjectivity, and avoiding multiculturalism, leading to authentic hybrid research and collaborative learning
4. Proactive stance, real action by empowered people, leading to prominence in search of alternatives to the lack of policies and public investments, subjects acting to protect themselves, and fighting for their rights

Still, on this last quoted text, the participatory cyclical processes can be carried out throughout a flow of participatory tools that enable direct participation of the subjects; a few examples of such tools are presented in Table 4.1 with a brief summary and references. Besides the ongoing process to be reflexive with regard on feedbacks, there are also alternative relevant interactions in the participatory processes making use of conventional scientific instruments and analytics. Such increments can be conceived as mediations (see Fig. 4.1) like samplings, environmental monitoring, epidemiological surveys, and own quantitative or qualitative analysis allowing the subjects to work together with the researchers. This kind of scientific inputs can enable a real collaborative work empowering subjects as researchers, or on the other hand, it can be a means for answering legitimate questions that come from the dialogical process. The application of conventional scientific tools can be considered as instruments of indirect participation, regardless of a significant power of promoting positive feedbacks in the dialogical process.

Table 4.1 Some participatory tools with the power of dialogical interaction

Participatory tool and reference	Summary
Talking map/sketch map (Toledo and Pelicioni 2009; Toledo and Giatti 2014)	Collective manual drawings representing subjects' contexts, to be produced by subgroups in a meeting. Participants are motivated by a leading question to discuss and work in collaboration. It is a very successful tool for initial contacts with groups opening dialog and initiating participation of people from communities, for example. At the end of the section, each one of the subgroups should make the produced map "to talk," that is to say a presentation for the whole group at the meeting, fostering discussion on the different views and discussions on the same question (see Figs. 4.2 and 4.3)
Photovoice (Findholt et al. 2011)	Involves the use of photography produced by the subjects in the sense of documenting, reflecting, and communicating on a common interest issue, and in this regard, photovoice can even provide the possibility for a dialog with policymakers strengthening engagement and a chance for social change. Subjects must produce photographs on a relevant issue, and then through workshops, it is possible to promote reflections and interactions
World café (Fouché and Light 2011)	A conversational activity to help groups to engage in collaborative dialog within critical questions. Through the application of leading questions on subgroups by hosts in different desks with questions to be answered. A process of pollination occurs when subjects (guests) exchange desks in successive rounds. A collective presentation made by hosts ends the dynamic, bringing the whole group to discuss. It is a powerful instrument for sharing information and fostering collaborative and equitable learning
River of life (Wallerstein et al. 2017a, b)	Applying the metaphor of a river, this is a tool to describe the life journey or any event in chronological order. Subjects are invited to organize into subgroups to describe an issue by the co-creation of a manual drawing through the conscious flowing description. It can be applied, for example, to describe the history of a community, or the "life" of the project, and the relationships with partnerships. Participants are also invited to a collective discussion on the drawings produced, and this is an appropriate tool for learning from each other and relating evolving processes
Venn diagrams (Mayoux 2001; Faridah Aini et al. 2017)	Participative elaboration of a social network representation associated with a given context or problem. It is useful to identify stakeholders and relationships as well as to find possible partnerships for collaboration. It can be made by a collective drawing or a scheme to be composed on the ground or even to be mounted in a wall, as in a communitarian space, then to be updated in the course of time. Different symbols or geometric shapes with respective meanings can be used, as well as relationships can be registered with the connections among different social actors. It is also useful to raise awareness on power relations and to identify the possibility to interact with relevant decisions through political engagement
Focus group (Gondim 2002; Rabiee 2004)	A technique for promoting group interactions on a topic suggested by the researcher and guided by a script of questions in similarity with an in-depth group interview. Participants are selected because of their domain on the studied issue or as representatives of the studied context. Focus groups can bring a range of ideas, feelings, and perspectives from individuals, thereby making possible collective reflection, dialog and collaborative learning, and production of answers for the applied questions. Also, it can be a resource for understanding the processes of perceptions building, taking action, and exploring social representations among human groups

(continued)

Table 4.1 (continued)

Participatory tool and reference	Summary
Culture circles (Moura and Lima 2014; Sampaio et al. 2014; Freire 2000)	Collective participation in debates through successive rounds in conversation circles on a certain issue in which it is possible to dialog with the subjects. In such a conversation, subjects express themselves and listen to others in a reflexive activity. The interactive process characterizes a cyclical investigation and an opportunity for educative liberation. This was a process of motivational experiences that grounded the development Paulo Freire's methodology dedicated to adult literacy (Freire 2018)
Community newspaper (Toledo et al. 2012)	Elaboration of a handcraft newspaper by a group of representatives of the studied issue or problem in a community. Participants must choose among different editorial positions to take part in the process of bringing reflexive contribution to the problem that must aggregate collective interests, surpassing the informative function of the product. The community newspaper can be an instrument for social action and transformation, by utilizing the participatory construction and by the process of disseminating the newspaper and discussing with the whole community on related concerns

Source: elaborated by the author

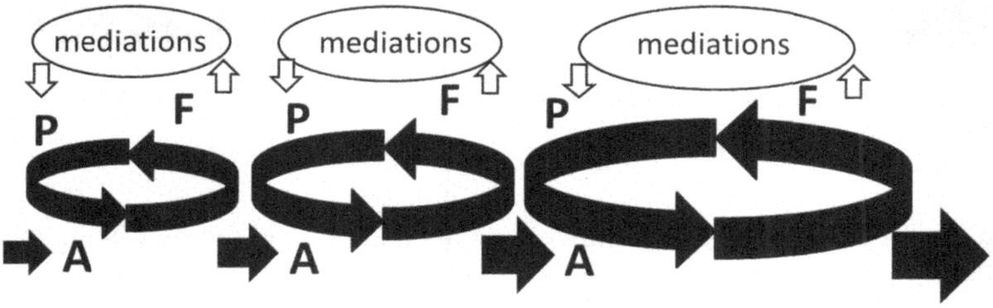

Fig. 4.1 Dialogical cyclical process of participatory research. Key: (P) - planning; (A) - action; (F) - feedback/fact-finding. Source: adapted from (Toledo and Giatti 2014)

The whole process of interaction should be open to dialog and continuous adaptation based on intersubjective outcomes and insights. Thus, to make a real dialogical interaction it is necessary to embody the process with democratic decisions regarding the subjects, and this sometimes can redirect the methodological procedures. That is one more point of necessary humility on behalf of the researchers, also conditioning the quality of sharing power with process feasibility.

There is an enormous variety of tools for applying in participatory research, and any compilation can exhaust the possibilities, even because creativity can be considered to expand alternatives and to promote adaptation of tools. The tools can be appropriately chosen on the conditions and objectives to pursue or on the characteristics of the group of subjects to be involved. Besides those presented in Table 4.1, many authors have contributed to the present compilations of useful instruments that can help to proceed with dialogical participatory projects and interventions.

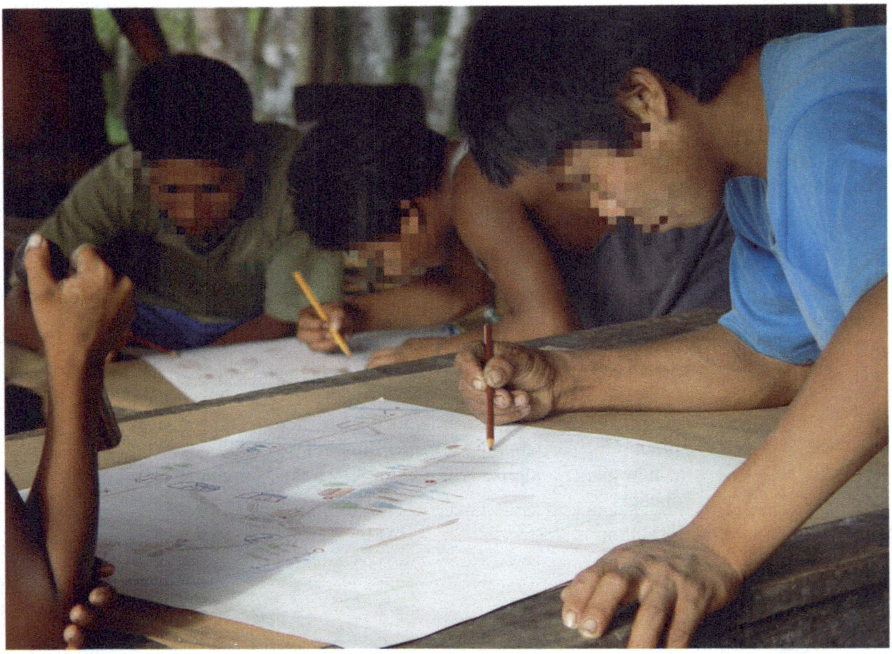

Fig. 4.2 Collective elaboration of a talking map in an indigenous community in Brazil. Source: the author

Lynam et al. (2007) in a review paper presents and depicts on the effectiveness of ten different tools that have been undertaken to incorporate community knowledge, preferences, and values into decision-making in the field of natural resources management. Among them, "participatory mapping" consists in developing representations of spatial relationships among real structures and objects captured by participants and converted into sketches. This tool can be considered as similar to the presented "talking maps" in Table 4.1, but it is worth to note that among the vast diversity of tools, similarities can be quite considerable.

Oettle et al. (2014) also bring a valuable contribution related to natural resources but specifically concerned with the perspective of climate change and local disturbances that require a robust community-based capacity of responses, adaptability, and resilience. The authors also compile several appropriate tools in this sense and among them the "climate diaries" that is based on the routine of registering subjects. perceptions and observations on the local climate-related phenomena, like maximum and minimum temperature, humidity, hours of sunshine, total rainfall, and extreme events. This tool allows people to build, share, and compare their records. Another valuable tool applicable to climate concerns is "participatory water monitoring" that can encompass collaborative identification of areas prone to severe water shortage in dry seasons, also jointly with planning of emergency and collective measures for attending to critical levels of water scarcity, for instance.

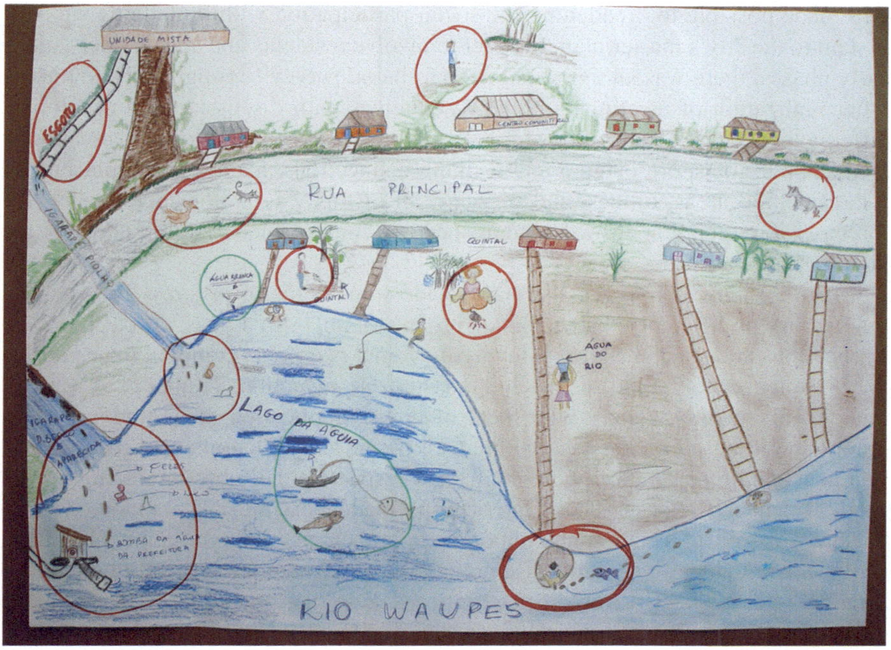

Fig. 4.3 Talking map elaborated on a leading question: what are "good" or "bad" things for health in the environment?—an indigenous community in Brazil. Note: The good things are circled in green and the bad in red. Source: the author

Participatory tools have also been applied to projects associated with the payment for environmental services and sustainability, considering the local concerns on environmental resources, economics, and social inclusion. In this sense, Faridah Aini et al. (2017) also provide an useful bundle of participatory tools dedicated to forestry and livelihoods research, like the "participatory rapid marked appraisal," that allows micro- and small-scale entrepreneurs to develop new products and to consider new customers as possible alternatives to manage forest resources and the asset of native fruit trees. Such a process allowed the consideration of gender and age-segregated groups in Malaysia, promoting freedom of expression and fostering social learning on ecological, organizational, and market-relevant aspects.

Although the objective of this book is to explore face-to-face dialogical activities, technological tools can provide insights, alternatives, and stimulate social actors to participate in activities, sometimes propitiating creativity and use of local resources and proper incentives for social mobilization. In this regard, participatory GIS can enhance the potential of community mapping as well as to making a bridge for social learning with support with a technological platform that conventionally is always in the domain of experts from academia or decision-making (de Carvalho and Giatti 2018). In Helsinki, Finland, an action research applied through participatory

GIS made possible to broadening the social participation within planning support system to the city's master plan. In order to involve residents and stakeholders since early phases, there was an initial online map-based survey (through website links). After realization of meetings with representatives with discussions on developed different geocoded visualizations for issues of interest like provision of recreational areas, public transport, cycling and walking connections, natural areas, placement for residential areas, offices, and services, all of this was in consideration of the forecast of population growth and respective consequences (Kahila-Tani et al. 2016).

Citizen science initiatives also have made some signs of progress in fostering interactions of different social actors on urban sustainability issues with technology applications and social networks. Involving young people on complex issues of the WEF (water, energy, food) nexus and disaster risk reduction, Trajber et al. (2019) made a mix methods study with local mapping, application of qualitative interviews, and the use of a bespoke mobile/cell phone "app" that allowed participants to a geocoded recording of photographs and respective daily life interactions with food, water, and energy. These interactions made possible the elaboration of a "visual web" of information and a looping approach enabling young people to co-analyze their data, co-learn, and also getting them closer to the possibility of appropriating issues related to urban planning and complex interactions, like climate change, sustainability, and their own quality of life. Also, an alternative to engage young people in a legitimate relationship with such issues that conventionally are addressed just through top-down schemes was enabled.

Besides the vast variety of tools for participatory research, there is also the possibility of adapting or merging some tools in order to find better conditions of application in consideration of the social group that is targeted, their literacy, and previous experiences with collaborative activities. In this sense, it is valid to ask: In such a frame of a diversity of tools, how about scientific rigor and quality in terms of reaching research objectives?

The answer to this question comes alongside the interpretation that participatory processes have no correspondence to the conventionally expected replicability because the whole interaction is ruled by intersubjectivity. Then, relevant criteria to follow must be the orientation of participatory research for intervention (action) and collaborative learning. For instance, Thiollent (2011) emphasizes that research action (*pesquisa-ação* in Portuguese) is characterized as empirical social research based on collaborative learning involving academics and subjects, working together in search of a possible resolution of a specific problem. For that matter, the scientific rigor must be oriented to a satisfactory production of narratives, within a process of good dialogical quality, social learning, and with progressive construction of alternatives and engagement with problem-solving on behalf of subjects' interest.

Such requisites can be much more challenging than just reproducing replicable tools and so, making necessarily great attention to the process that will be permeated the intersubjectivity and the circumstance of sharing the power of choice with the subjects on the direction of the research process. The dialogical nature of interactions represents a real engagement with the recognition that subjects' expectations are relevant to build trust, and their perspectives on the appropriation of the research project will be determining of genuine symmetrical cooperation and co-production of hybrid knowledge. Otherwise, sometimes it will not be easy to attain a legitimate dialogical interaction when following the same direction of solving the selected initial problem. Therefore, it always remains the constant trade-off on these two dimensions of rigor in participatory research: the building and maintenance of a legitimate dialogical interaction as sharing power, and the direction of creating a collaborative pathway for action and problem-solving.

These considerations are much more related to the participatory process as a full flow instead of just to the quality of any employed participatory tool. The process will be the sequence of participatory tools applied, but always having in mind the extended results to reach, as the collaborative learning and searching for alternatives, the symmetrical interactions, and the perspectives of sharing power as to empowering people that many times are in a disadvantaged and vulnerable condition. That is a crucial aspect of proceeding with evolving mutual interactions through the application of participatory tools in a cyclical dynamic. Such a proceeding must be skilled to learn and adapt in consideration of a good quality of dialogical participation. Figure 4.1 presents the dynamics of the cyclical participatory process, which includes aspects of growing dialogicity, trust, reciprocity, and empowerment. The expected increase of such attributes is represented by the expansion of the cycles in the scheme, in reference to the process evolution carried out by ongoing actions (A), feedbacks (F—also for fact-finding), and planning (P).

The progress of participatory dialogical interactions must enable insights and demands that were not previously conceived because they result from the intersubjectivity and the cultural background of the subjects. In that way, some questionings can emerge, for example, requiring application of traditional scientific tools, as mentioned above. Besides, such demands can be related to the need to bring a different specialist to the community or to provide a course or workshop to create new local capacities. Also, such insights and demands can come as the realization of cultural activity, or a bazaar, as in the related case in Guarulhos to get cash for implementing the community garden (Chap. 3). All of these supplements to the process can be seen as mediations, and so, they show relevance in strengthening trust and reciprocity, also increasing social mobilization and legitimate engagement.

The flow of the process can be carried out in, at least, two distinct forms: the first, by combining participatory tools, like those presented in Table 4.1; second, by the development of collaborative research with the involvement of subjects in the phases of research like planning, defining and applying methods, and analyzing evidence. For participatory processes carried by participatory tools, conventional research tools (like environmental analysis, surveys) can come as mediations, thus responding to legitimate concerns of the subjects. For those processes conducted by collaborative research, distinct participatory tools can assume the role of mediations, also with the power of immediate and active participation, but promoting reflection and intersubjectivity in the flow of the research development.

As a system of interactions, the participatory process can be understood as a living organism. Anyhow, besides the metaphor, the participatory process in its adaptability assumes an autopoietic property. Thus, it is vital that researchers be sensitive and apprehend such a feature. The process self-organizes through subjects' interactions and actions on the concrete reality, then changing itself into something different (a more robust dialogical process) in each round, increasing its desirable ongoing outcomes. The process regulating itself relates to the health of the interaction, something that must be constantly diagnosed and strengthened. Taking care of the health of the participatory process on behalf of the researchers means systematically analyzing feedbacks of the ongoing interactions. Then it relates to analyzing and solving possible conflicts, establishing co-habitation rules and ways of sharing possible benefits, attending to legitimate demands from the subjects, and building and maintaining trust.

Also, a CBPR framework presented by Kastelic et al. (2017) can help in keeping attention to the health of the process, as well as to planning or continuously evaluating the projects. That is a very flexible and adaptive framework, which consists of organizing the approach into four overarching domains: contexts, partnership processes, intervention and research, and outcomes. The model assumes the hypothesis that in any context of application, community-academic partnership grounds the partnership processes, those that will be the essence of engagement to affect and alter the "science" or the design of intervention and research. The application of this model can occur in a workshop involving researchers and subjects, and they can orient the process to the search for desired outcomes, then analyzing contexts, partnerships, and necessary interventions. On the other hand, the same model can be applied for planning and evaluating a participatory research process in successive moments, like before, during, and after the implementation of any project.

In combining different tools, sometimes researchers repeat the same tools many times; however, it can occur also by evaluating the quality of the process of interaction with particular benefits and outputs. In fact, there is a prime concern on the quality and the intent of the chosen tool. For example, focus groups started to be applied in the first half of the twentieth century, mainly for understanding the reactions of subjects to propaganda, or in the marketing field or related to organizational development. Of course, there is no problem in applying focus groups to these segments, but sometimes this kind of practice can be much more committed to the company's interests than to the subjects' needs and wishes.

However, in the sense of an application of focus group in a participatory process that searches for empowerment, collaboration, and symmetrical relationships, the quality criteria of this tool must be attached to the quality of process in order for it to be dialogical. Actually, in this sense focus groups can be adequately qualified for participatory processes because of their power to aggregate distinguishable worldviews helping to build awareness on common issues, and their perspective of fostering collective changes of mindsets and behaviors (Tanaka and Santana 2018). Among varieties of applications for this same tool, an intervention research held in Brazil on perceptions of risks of climate change and adaptation strategies made use of following focus groups on collectives of researchers, practitioners and policymakers, neighborhood leaders, and young people. This particular application among different groups showed the possible interactive process as to demonstrate a possibility to spread the intervention within different stakeholders who are implied in risky contexts (Serrao-Neumann et al. 2013).

4.3 Integrating Uncertainties

Again on the distinctive nature of participatory research and its methodological flexibility and self-organizing adaptive feature: does it seem to be too expensive an exchange? The decision on proceeding with participatory research concerning its requisites seems to make waver on the decision of leaving the safety and autonomy of those traditional methodologies traced by objectivity and replicability. That is something to be a contentious concern mainly for those who are deciding on a participatory approach for the first time. Nonetheless, the decision of proceeding with participatory research is not a matter of choosing an alternative method; indeed, this is a decision on what kind of interaction with society the researcher wants to build. Moreover, it indicates the researcher's decision in recognition that he or she is interested in learning with the subjects, and then it shows something relevant to find more sophisticated arrangements to deal with complex issues. Participatory approaches are not better than, nor comparable with, traditional methods of research. Actually, participatory research is complementary to the relationship of academics with society, and in this regard, its objectives can be distinguishable by the collaborative results to be attained through dialogical interactions, empowerment, and a myriad of outcomes associated with the participatory process.

Also, within this nature of dynamical and reciprocal relationships, the loss of autonomy begins to make sense in a relevant and urgent flow for a new social contract with science. Such a context has been inherently characterized, for example, as the way that society sometimes has fought to get prominence in the quality control demarcation for scientific statements that raise controversies (Gibbons 1999). From this point of view, in which society must be naturally questioning the scientific production and respective high risks of consequences as emergent and unpredictable side effects, participatory research seems to be a brave and legitimate choice.

In regard to post-normal problems, there is one more worthy value of participatory research in the context of emergent complexities. Participatory approaches as being welcoming to more open and adaptive interactions are also receptive of uncertainty. Indeed, it is remarkable that researchers in doing participatory research are obligated to follow the problems wherever they adopt the interactive process (Brydon-Miller et al. 2003). Thus, although before we thought that missing the absolute control of the methods would be a high deprivation, now we can conceive that the proceeding of sharing power and being open to new forms of organization of the process (or even a legitimate self-organization in dialogical relationships with the subjects) can make possible an open structure to bring uncertainties into the method, indeed, at the core of the intersubjective interaction.

There is an appropriate analogy in this concern, as post-normal science stresses the centeredness of uncertainty. In the dilemma of assuming the limits of "normal science," good quality of information is dependent on recognition and proper management of its uncertainties. For that matter, post-normal problems require systemic and humanistic methods to incorporate dialog between stakeholders and scientists on systemic uncertainties, and collective decision on multiple stakes to guide appropriate problem-solving strategies (Funtowicz and Ravetz 1993).

The unpredictability of complex issues encounters equivalence in the method that begins as open to uncertainty in its own development. In this kind of participatory processes with a flexible and adaptive structure, uncertainty finds correspondence and acceptance instead of negligence. As stated before, uncertainties and ambivalence were always banished by modern science. The cyclical and reflexive interactions are fundamental for recognizing uncertainties from a democratic perspective, also embracing the intrinsic ambivalence from different points of view and values. With participatory research, there is an innovative way of incorporating the challenging and sometimes intentionally forgotten uncertainties and ambivalence, and this can make a different scope to reinforce the importance of opting for such an approach.

4.4 Meta-Information in Participatory Research

Qualitative empirical research has the power to produce in-depth explanations about the nature of problems subordinated to social dimensions. In contrast to quantitative methods that focus on the objectivity of data, good sampling designs, and sophisticated statistical analysis for exploring causal links, qualitative research dedicates to go further in clarifications on why those variables in causal analysis can be associated. In this sense, qualitative approaches explore narratives and a myriad of explanations of phenomena, including some of those that can be concealed from the researchers' eyes.

The argument here is that in comparison with conventional qualitative research approaches, participatory ones allow maximizing the power of explanation and also foster creating and producing new reflexive information associated with the intersubjective process of collaborative aggregation of different knowledges.

With the ongoing social learning feature, participatory approaches also bring opportunity for the emergence of innovative hybrid explanations and alternatives, new meanings, and interpretations of phenomena. The creative and reflexive asset of participatory research also induces the production of something that I have considered on the designation of "meta-information."

The Greek prefix *meta* refers to attributes of transcendence, change, and also the means of self-reflection. Thus, meta-information in participatory approaches can transcend as being produced and registered in the intersection of knowledges separated by the conventional rupture of cognitive exclusion. Accordingly, it can be related to change in a reflexive perspective. For instance, community social actors when working together in a participatory tool application can have a unique opportunity to put their particular understandings to build different collective and robust new understandings, sometimes making possible the emergence of disruptive conceptions or questionings. Even the interaction of community members on a specific issue can make possible the appearance of data that would be unexpected within individual focus. Such processes and affluence of meta-information are not natural to occur in normal conditions as in scenarios of low social mobilization, or in circumstances of little perception of important collective problems, low self-esteem, and lack of empowerment.

Meta-information is related to transcendence, reflection, and dialogical interaction among the subjects and can be registered by the researchers with incremental power for apprehending complexity. Sometimes, it can also be useful to evaluate the quality of the dialogical interactions. Moreover, it can be associated with the production of meta-knowledge, as Avenier et al. (1999, p. 66) describes a category of "knowledge constructed over the course of the research process about the overall organization," in the case of the application of intervention research bringing together parties involved in finding organizational solutions.

Besides, meta-information can be recognized as a pattern of meta-data, in other words, related to data about data (Higgins 1999), like regarding data contents, format, context, quality, structure, and accessibility (Michener 2006). In that direction, the association with a participatory research process the meta-information can bring accounts on information at the basis of how the socio-ecological system operates, also describing essential elements like who, what, when, where, and how, everything in regard to the reflexive interactions among social actors. Therefore, such meta-information can emerge in the process and thus, it can be useful to identify the source quality and the credibility of the information that has been produced to answer the straight questions on the investigation. For example, if we are working collaboratively with urban community members on relating the history of the neighborhood creation, then a kind of meta-information can be the understanding about how people involved are legitimate to tell an authentic history (Higgins 1999). This legitimization of information can occur in the collective narrative production through the subjects' interactions and trust building, then generating plenty of qualitative evidence to the researcher.

Also, it can be worthy to explore relations of power and knowledge in a community or within a process of interaction among social actors with different attributes, like age, gender, literacy, income, or hierarchy. The refinement in the acquisition of information on the interaction can provide valuable information to care about the health of the participatory process. For example, distinguishable asymmetries concerning hierarchy can be identified and managed to avoid tensions or ruptures towards the participants.

To make a pragmatic description, it is worth to consider some fieldwork experiences. In the participatory approach held in Iauaretê, Brazilian Amazon, an adaptation of a photovoice (photo panel) helped to diagnose some relevant insights (Toledo and Giatti 2014). Indigenous people were previously mobilized to take pictures of their local livelihoods, registering relevant environmental aspects on health and disease. After with photos in the paper, they were invited to describe in panels causes,

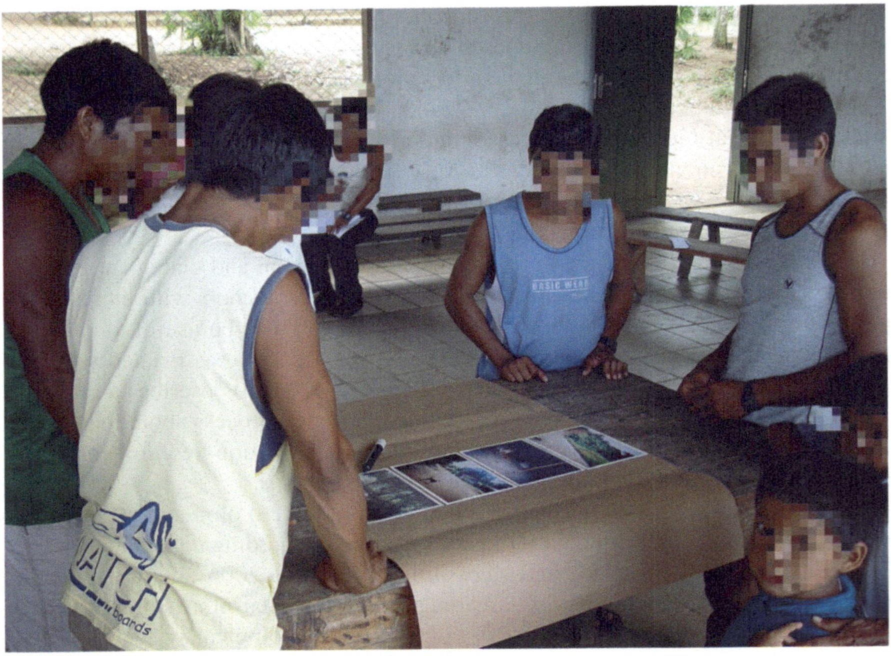

Fig. 4.4 Mounting photo panels in Iauaretê, describing causes and consequences for problems related in pictures. Source: the author

and possible solutions to the problems showed by their own pictures (see Fig. 4.4). Spontaneously, when making presentations about the developments for the whole group in the workshops (Fig. 4.5), the subjects conducted their conversation about problems, causes, and possible solutions in Tukano language, the most popular local language. They speak Portuguese regularly, but mostly to talk to "white people" and in institutions, like the local school, local army base, and church. The researchers chose to talk among themselves in Tukano as an indicative of common interest in having a conversation to address those local relevant problems. The ongoing development of the workshop corroborated it, since after their own reflections, there were volunteer explanations in Portuguese addressed to the researchers because they did not have the domain of Tukano. This arrangement was a pattern on the sequential repetition of the photo panel in 10 local community centers in Iauaretê, as the methodology of the research project proceeded.

In this case, some circumstances allowed considering the production and registering of relevant meta-information. For instance, the attitude of speaking in Tukano was in that direction, then showing the quality of subjects' involvement in the discussion. Such behavior denoted a social mobilization on the issue. It occurred transcending the process of acquiring the information intended by the participatory tool applied, which was their narratives about causes and possible solutions for sanitary problems. The quality of debate appropriation also was corroborated by the historical

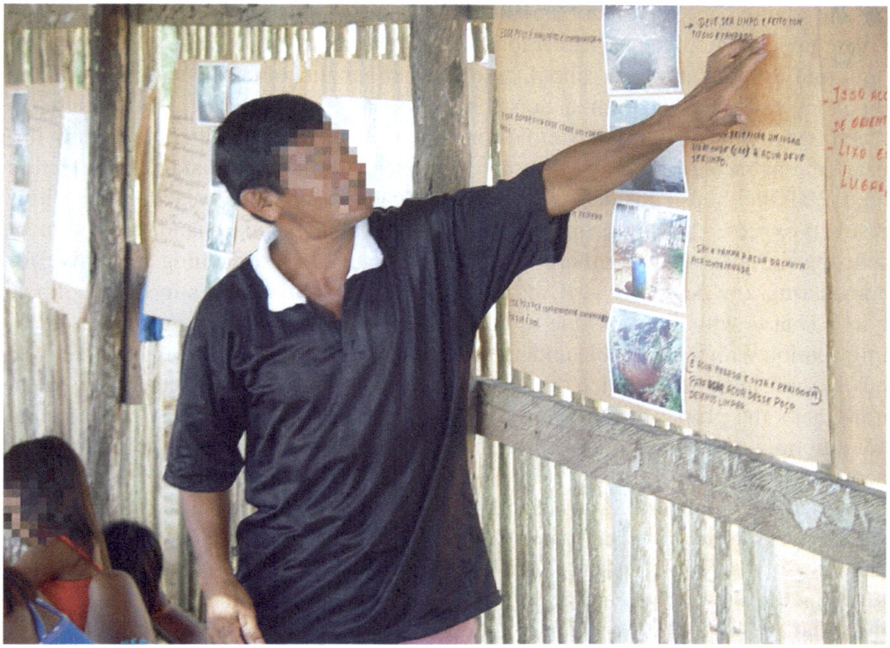

Fig. 4.5 Presenting and discussing the concerns in photo panels, interacting with the community on their own problems and reflections. Source: the author

relationship of indigenous of that region with the surrounding society, since they have a traditional protocol to interact with people of institutions, also keeping a social position called "capitão," just to proceed with these conversations. Similarly, the following attitude of explaining the previous conversation in Portuguese to the researchers brought more meta-information associated with trust and reciprocity concerning researchers that were from outside the community.

Another unusual situation to be related was carried out in the ResNexus project (see Chap. 3), working with young people in Guarulhos municipality, Brazil. When developing a talking map, the young participants were asked to sketch with the purpose of planning possible and desired improvements to the Novo Recreio neighborhood in Guarulhos. It was an exercise of approximation with urban planning in a frame of 5 years with the acquisition of data for composing the Participatory GIS. As regular in this kind of participatory tool, subgroups of about 5–6 young participants were developing their cardboard designs for the sequence of collective presentation and reflection. Then, a relevant statement emerged systematically from the subgroups, which was like "I will not be living here within 5 years." That was a claim full of meanings and perceptions, which had not been stated necessarily to answer to the applied question on planning improvements 5 years ahead.

The claim was very natural and spoken among their conversations as being young people who live in a vulnerable and peripheral urban community, deprived of opportunities, leisure, high school, among other benefits of urban centers. In telling this, they showed to recognize their conditions and the lack of local possibilities to reach a standard of living desirable for young people. In such a context, they finished the process of planning desirable benefits and made a satisfactory reflection on the talking maps considering feasible alternatives, as well as reaching a positive result as expected by the participatory tool applied. On the other hand, the statement refusing the idea of living there for 5 years remained as something restrictive for considering any perspective of searching for substantive changes in the neighborhood. That is why it is possible to consider this spontaneous statement as a meta-information with the valuable understanding that goes beyond the primal objectives, but has intrinsic importance as a determinant of the context. Such a statement transcends the proposed reflection and also, at the same time, shows fundamental conditioning that could become hidden, but emerge in the legitimate space of interaction among the subjects.

Researchers must be sensitive and prepared to capture meta-information, which can have a significant value to explore the potential of participatory research with elements of reflection, learning, and empowerment. However, it sounds that sometimes meta-information emerges almost silently or between the lines of the narratives that are produced. Most important, researchers must be attentive to the process of interaction among subjects, always registering any possible relevant manifestations or insights.

Still, in comparison with participatory research, other qualitative social approaches can provide different information and explanations about those studied phenomena. Then, joining narratives from different social actors can provide a diversity of valuable data, through subjects' knowledge, expertise, and points of view. For example, interviewing people on the relevance of climate change and health-related effects can result in a broad range of perceptions in consideration of applying to people of different countries, with different backgrounds or even supposed to be in different conditions of vulnerability due to multifactorial, climate, and health-related risks (Akerlof et al. 2010). With such an amount of data, it is possible, for instance, to compare distinct perceptions or also to encounter various understandings on the relation of climate change and health consequences.

However, it is regularly possible to reach a sum of those diversified perceptions and explanations. Analyzing the creative possibilities and accurately dedicating on participatory approaches, it is possible to confirm that the dialogical interactions result in something much more productive than a sum of pieces, since in the process of collaborative and reflexive learning "A" plus "B" can be AB and also a myriad of new meanings, reflections, and understandings.

Because of the ordinary negligence of uncertainties in the normal production of scientific statements, decision-making is also induced to conceal doubts and small or not well-estimated possibilities of failure (Funtowicz and Ravetz 1993; Ravetz 2004). When a debate involving different stakeholders occurs, as in an induced participatory interaction, it comes to disclose elements of doubt, risks, and uncertainties, and then a legitimate condition of questioning the relationship science-decision-making emerges as a response to the conventional ruptures that isolate social actors from the debate.

The questioning process in this sense can be related to ascertaining the quality of scientific discourse production, in terms of searching for uncertainties, ambiguity, and risks of mistakes and failures in decisions. In that way, meta-information can be understood as characteristics or qualifiers of information that can affect the accurateness of decision, with a possible association with aspects of the processing and communicating the information or also situational awareness of the relevance of the variables involved (Pfautz et al. 2006). For instance, some possible questioning can be like: who studied, who funded, and how was the scientific proof produced? Alternatively, another questioning can be: what is the credible comparison between a guinea pig in a laboratory and a human being living in an urban environment to evaluate the limits for particular substance exposure? All of these and similar questions gain status of meta-information and legitimacy along the intersubjective interactions.

More than empowering people trough debating and having protagonism within decisions, this legitimate attitude of promoting participatory approaches helps to overcome the cognitive exclusion that keeps uncertainties and high stakes concealed with the possibility of systemic and emergent damages. In this regard, the appearance of contestation in such democratic debate relates to the need for meta-information as debriefing on qualifying factors of the scientific statements, and then it makes the applicability of participatory research on post-normal problems valuable. On the other hand, that is also related to knowledge democratization that implies in sharing power on taking decisions based on scientific statements that can encompass doubts, ignorance, or even conflicting interests. Notably, the cyclical and dialogical process of successive interactions involving different social actors can be understood as liberating from the oppressive context in which laypersons cannot contest scientific hegemony. However, as those laypersons have their stakes, so they also must have the power to argue on decisions permeated by severe risks. Meta-information, as identified, seems to play a role in denoting the strength of such a reflexive and dialogical participatory process.

4.5 The Process as a Product

The characteristic of merging objectives of intervention and investigation gives participatory research a variety of possible outcomes. As in researching, it is possible to answer scientific questions as well proceed with hypothesis testing. However, the meaning of investigating/researching also brings the perspective of mutual learning among different social actors to be involved in participatory interactions searching for changes. In turn of the systemic interactions provided by the cyclical and dialogical interactions, the chance of achieving concrete outcomes and empowerment expands by the possibilities aggregated or created in the process, like as finding or enhancing partnerships, exploring the creative role of social practices, or even as with the multiplier stance of the ecology of knowledge.

Kurt Lewin with his contributions on action research applied to improve organizational structures by involving different parties also delimitated aspects of multiple gains of interventions, as so, the change-inducing targeting runs alongside the process of researching one of the various forms of social action (Lewin 1947). Following other organizational appliances of action research, Avenier et al. (1999) emphasize that there can be a process of negotiation among the social actors as different interest parties. Then cross-fertilization between their possible different projects can result in another project that will be common to both parties, to be constructed as an advance in an ongoing process of constructivist conception of knowledge. This collaborative progress can bring disruptive effects for the intervention on organizations, and can produce varied forms of knowledge, some of which can be publishable in the sense of scientific production of papers, and others that can be a local knowledge of interest and applicability on the studied case. As the last, meta-knowledge - as the subjects appropriate of meta-information and - also arises in the process, offering relevant information produced and apprehended by the participants, having a fundamental role in describing attributes of the system in study and intervention.

The perspective of joining distinct interests can even be associated with the multifunctional nature of participatory research. However, in the sense of the Freirian proposals, liberation from oppression must also be taken into account as a goal to be targeted, mainly in consideration of the existence of oppressive relationships. In this concern, liberation in parallel with empowerment can also be a result of participatory processes as with the ongoing evolution of methods and the search for solving common problems (Wallerstein et al. 2017a, b; Freire 2000).

The ongoing collaborative knowledge production through participatory processes to address sustainability can engender dimensions of social learning that can also represent a relationship with distinct outcomes per se. For that matter, Wildemeersch (2007) exposes four dimensions of interrelated activities: the first is "social action" that can operate through needs and competencies presented in the social system involved, which is a means of engaging people in solving a common problem; the second is related to "reflection" and is triggered by social learning as the collective making of balances, questioning processes, norms, and values, also encompassing rational and emotional aspects; third is "communication" that can occur as a product and a benefit both inside and outside of the approached social system; and the last dimension is "negotiation" on differences of interest and limitations of the system, also interplaying between inside and outside actors and factors.

Participatory research can be seen as a work in progress, continually challenging positivist as embracing a notion of knowledge as socially constructed. The nature of working collaboratively with other social actors leads not only to community and organizational changes but also to personal changes for subjects and for the researcher. Some changes for the researcher must be with the need to reinterpret the act of researching in a different notion of objective and the surpassing of the idea of value-free approach, since deciding on proceeding with intervention means at an explicit political choice. The acceptance of values leads to the imperative of action, and in turn, knowledge emerges from doing, from the initiatives. The democratic practice of a socially engaged research sets the context in which value-free cannot be proceeded as in natural science, and the decision on it is itself a change, but the process of change for the researcher is a rule in the ongoing development of action research (Brydon-Miller et al. 2003).

Since the process of finding generative themes with the subjects, and fostering respective coding and decoding situations, there is a reflection and production of new and collaborative knowledge. The emergence of knowledge and aggregated information, of great interest for the researchers and the subjects, means at the process as connections of the subjects' concrete world with the academic assumptions or with the perspective of policymakers. Information and knowledge transcend the relation with the problem on approach, creating bridges and approximations with particular support for cognitive inclusion and ecology of knowledge. At the same, the social learning development as a reciprocal and negotiated process contributes to finding and fostering partnerships including local competences. It leads to empowerment as well as making possible advocacy in regard to vulnerable people. The realization of vulnerable people in navigating to other scales and interacting with institutions in itself makes a singular output.

Like a process of ongoing teaching by learning and learning by teaching (Freire 2000) in participatory research, a context permeated by ignorance and uncertainty compels academics, policymakers, and subjects to continuously learn, teach, and reflect as pursuing changes by action on the concrete world. In this regard, participatory research processes have a generator potential of creative answers, knowledges, and actions.

At the beginning of a participatory research project, the researcher begins from a fragmented view of the context and related problems. Only with a dialogical interaction, there can be an opportunity to apprehend the reality from the point of view of the subjects, something that must be considered as relevant to conditioning vulnerabilities, for instance. In addition, as acquiring the notion that the world just can be understood by trying to change it (Brydon-Miller et al. 2003), we are obligated to recognize that the nature of current problems related to inequities, unsustainability, and health concerns can be associated with the fragmentation of social groups, on their knowledges and practices. In this regard, the perspective of reaching social inclusion with cognitive justice must be a horizon to research as performing collaborative engagements trying to change the contexts. Only in such processes with dialogical interactions it is possible to expect the emergence of hybrid knowledge good enough to explain the complexities and also able to be apprehended by different social actors, like subjects of vulnerable contexts, policymakers, and researchers.

The problems threatening humankind were never so connected, interdependent and with the perspective of such fast dissemination, disruptive and emergent side effects, and systemic consequences. The contemporary problems are also permeated by a high level of uncertainties and contradictions, as related to varied value judgments and respective social tensions and struggles. The changing world order is ongoing with no possible conventional interpretation, for instance, a volcanic eruption in Iceland in 2010 caused chaos in the European airline traffic, and this kind of event can quickly call the world's attention, inducing other possibilities of effects as by the economic burden of intrinsic operations (Sardar 2015). Maybe it is time for finding back the properties of our powerful natural ability to coupling as to make more valuable our diversities of knowledges, creativity, and practices. As discussed before, the rupture characterized by cognitive exclusion inhibits possible interactions and ecologies of knowledges that would give a chance to a myriad of alternatives and subjects insertions in collaborative structures. Thus, systems of interactions through dialogical participatory research should be understood through this property of recovering our capacities for more interaction. Also, this is a liberation from oppression and ruptures that inhibit our self-organizing competences.

Considering the diversity of outcomes in participatory research, it is worthy to recognize that the participatory processes can represent a product itself. A prominent analogy in that direction is valid: the participatory process is at the same time producer and the product itself, in accordance with the autopoiesis concept. Moreover, such a production can be multiple and varied, as bringing action and transforming social contexts, allowing dialogical interactions and collaborative ongoing knowledge, enabling necessary negotiations, empowering people, overcoming abyssal cognitive exclusion, providing conditions for the emergence of reflexive scientific evidence, and also fostering constant changes and learning for different social actors, including researchers.

References

Akerlof, K., DeBono, R., Berry, P., et al. (2010). Public perceptions of climate change as a human health risk: Surveys of the United States, Canada and Malta. *International Journal of Environmental Research and Public Health, 7*, 2559–2606.

Avenier, M.-J., Nourry, L., & Sweeney, M. (1999). Sciences of the artificial and knowledge production: The crucial role of intervention research in management sciences. *Design Issues, 15*, 55–70.

Baum, F. E. (2016). Power and glory: Applying participatory action research in public health. *Gaceta Sanitaria, 30*, 405–407.

Brydon-Miller, M., Greenwood, D., & Maguire, P. (2003). *Why action research?* London: Sage Publications.

Cargo, M., & Mercer, S. L. (2008). The value and challenges of participatory research: Strengthening its practice. *Annual Review of Public Health, 29*, 325–350.

de Carvalho, C. M., & Giatti, L. L. (2018). Participatory GIS for urban sustainability and resilience: A perspective of social learning and ecology of knowledge. In *Lifelong learning and education in healthy and sustainable cities* (pp. 21–34). Berlin: Springer.

Faridah Aini, M., Elias, M., Lamers, H., et al. (2017). Evaluating the usefulness and ease of use of participatory tools for forestry and livelihoods research in Sarawak, Malaysia. *Forests, Trees and Livelihoods, 26*, 29–46.

Findholt, N. E., Michael, Y. L., & Davis, M. M. (2011). Photovoice engages rural youth in childhood obesity prevention. *Public Health Nursing, 28*, 186–192.

Fouché, C., & Light, G. (2011). An invitation to dialogue: 'The world Café' in social work research. *Qualitative Social Work, 10*, 28–48.

Freire, P. (2000). *Pedagogy of the oppressed* (30th anniversary ed.) (M. B. Ramos, Trans., D. Macedo, Intro.) New York City: The Continuum International Publishing Group Inc.

Freire, A. M. A. (2018). *Paulo Freire: uma história de vida*. Editora Paz e Terra.

Funtowicz, S. O., & Ravetz, J. R. (1993). Science for the post-normal age. *Futures, 25*, 739–755.

Gibbons, M. (1999). Science's new social contract with society. *Nature, 402*, C81.

Gondim, S. M. G. (2002). Grupos focais como técnica de investigação qualitativa: desafios metodológicos. *Paidéia (Ribeirão Preto), 12*, 149–161.

Higgins, M. (1999). Meta-information, and time: Factors in human decision making. *Journal of the American Society for Information Science, 50*, 132–139.

Kahila-Tani, M., Broberg, A., Kyttä, M., & Tyger, T. (2016). Let the citizens map—Public participation GIS as a planning support system in the Helsinki master plan process. *Planning Practice & Research, 31*, 195–214.

Kastelic, S. L., Wallerstein, N., Duran, B., & Oetzel, J. G. (2017). Socio-ecologic framework for CBPR. In *Community-based participatory research for health: Advancing social and health equity* (p. 77).

Klinke, A., & Renn, O. (2012). Adaptive and integrative governance on risk and uncertainty. *Journal of Risk Research, 15*, 273–292.

Lewin, K. (1946). Action research and minority problems. *Journal of Social Issues, 2*, 34–46.

Lewin, K. (1947). Frontiers in group dynamics: II. Channels of group life; social planning and action research. *Human Relations, 1*, 143–153.

List, D. (2006). Action research cycles for multiple futures perspectives. *Futures, 38*, 673–684.

Lynam, T., De Jong, W., Sheil, D., et al. (2007). A review of tools for incorporating community knowledge, preferences, and values into decision making in natural resources management. *Ecology and Society, 12*(1), 5.

Maturana, H.R., Varela, F.J., (1992). The tree of knowledge (rev. ed.). Boston: Shambala.

Mayoux, L. (2001). *Participatory methods*. EDIAIS Application Guidance Note.

Michener, W. K. (2006). Meta-information concepts for ecological data management. *Ecological Informatics, 1*, 3–7.

Moura, A. F., & Lima, M. G. (2014). A Reinvenção da Roda: Roda de Conversa, um instrumento metodológico possível. *Revista Temas em Educação, 23*, 95–103.

Oettle, N., Koelle, B., Law, S., et al. (2014). *Participatory adaptation handbook: A practitioner's guide for facilitating people centered adaptation*. Cape Town, South Africa: Indigo Development & Change.

Pfautz, J., Roth, E., Bisantz, A., et al. (2006). *The role of meta-information in C2 decision-support systems*. Cambridge, MA: Charles River Analytics.

Rabiee, F. (2004). Focus-group interview and data analysis. *Proceedings of the Nutrition Society, 63*, 655–660.

Ravetz, J. (2004). The post-normal science of precaution. *Futures, 36*, 347–357.

Sampaio, J., Santos, G. C., Agostini, M., & Salvador, A. d. S. (2014). Limites e potencialidades das rodas de conversa no cuidado em saúde: uma experiência com jovens no sertão pernambucano. *Interface-Comunicação, Saúde, Educação, 18*, 1299–1311.

San Sebastián, M., & Hurtig, A. K. (2005). Oil development and health in the Amazon basin of Ecuador: The popular epidemiology process. *Social Science & Medicine, 60*, 799–807.

Sardar, Z. (2010). Welcome to postnormal times. *Futures, 42*, 435–444. https://doi.org/10.1016/j.futures.2009.11.028.

Sardar, Z. (2015). Postnormal times revisited. *Futures, 67*, 26–39.

Serrao-Neumann, S., Di Giulio, G. M., Ferreira, L. C., & Choy, D. L. (2013). Climate change adaptation: Is there a role for intervention research? *Futures, 53*, 86–97.

Tanaka, L. H., & Santana, C. L. A. (2018). Grupo focal como importante ferramenta de pesquisa participativa em saúde. In R. F. de Toledo et al. (Eds.), *Pesquisa Participativa em Saúde: Vertentes e Veredas*. São Paulo: Instituto de Saúde.

Thiollent, M. (2011). *Metodologia da Pesquisa-Ação* (18th ed.). São Paulo: Cortez.

Toledo, R. F., & Giatti, L. L. (2014). Challenges to participation in action research. *Health Promotion International, 30*, 162–173.

Toledo, R., & Pelicioni, M. (2009). A educação ambiental e a construção de mapas-falantes em processo de pesquisa-ação em comunidade indígena na Amazônia. *Revista Interacções, 5*, 193–213.

Toledo, R. F. d., Giatti, L. L., & Pelicioni, M. C. F. (2012). Social mobilization in health and sanitation in an action research process in an indigenous community in northwestern amazon. *Saúde e Sociedade, 21*, 206–218.

Trajber, R., Walker, C., Marchezini, V., et al. (2019). Promoting climate change transformation with young people in Brazil: Participatory action research through a looping approach. *Action Research, 17*, 87–107.

Wallerstein, N., Duran, B., Minkler, M., & Oetzel, J. G. (2017a). *Community-based participatory research for health: Advancing social and health equity*. Hoboken, NJ: Wiley.

Wallerstein, N., Giatti, L. L., Bógus, C. M., et al. (2017b). Shared participatory research principles and methodologies: Perspectives from the USA and Brazil—45 years after Paulo Freire's "Pedagogy of the oppressed". *Societies, 7*, 6.

Wildemeersch, D. (2007). Social learning revisited: Lessons learned from north and south. In *Social learning towards a more sustainable world* (pp. 99–116).

Chapter 5
The Need for a Taxonomy

5.1 A Diversity of Contexts, Approaches, and Purposes

The range of options and the self-organizing feature of participatory research approaches denote infinitude of applications, and within each one of the trials, the emergence of respective outcomes multiplicity. As stated before, the assortment of applications and the perspective of non-replicability of methods do not speak against the scientific rigor of participatory research, which must be oriented to the satisfactory production of narratives in terms of evidence production. Also, scientific rigor can be understood concerning the dialogical progress of interaction among different social actors involved, keeping in mind the pursuing of aims of change and the legitimate production of narratives based on symmetrical relationships, engagement, empowerment, collaborative learning, and knowledge production.

Stakeholder or subjects participation is an attribute substantially present at least as a recommendation to deal with sustainability and health promotion. Anyhow, sometimes participation can even be interpreted as a buzzword or just a recommendation at the end of texts that explore intertwined problems of socio-ecological systems. As a broad concept, participation involves practical, theoretical, and institutional senses, and it is just such multidimensionality and polysemy that incur in valuing and recognizing respective quality and effects, those that can be desirable or not.

The breadth of pathways for participatory research and the redirections due to the legitimate engagement of social actors seem to ascribe a degree of chaos, uncertainty, and messiness (Brydon-Miller et al. 2003). However, it is not detrimental as worsening the quality of research and intervention; it is about qualifying the plasticity and the adaptive property of such collaborative and integrated approaches.

To help understand possibilities, diversity, and multiplicity of purposes for participatory research, it is fundamental to discuss and characterize taxonomic elements to support signs of progress and to identify key challenges for those committed

L. L. Giatti, *Participatory Research in the Post-Normal Age*,
https://doi.org/10.1007/978-3-030-27924-0_5

with socio-transformation or concerned with socio-ecological sustainability transitions. Another relevant question in the myriad of alternatives and challenges is how to envisage participatory approaches as dealing with the sustainable and health issues that have causal chains operating through different scales from global to local. Taxonomic contributions in that way can help to make better choices related to the interests of researchers and subjects and the breadth of changes that can be attained.

In this chapter, there is the expectative to contribute to analyzing experiences and scientific bibliographic production about cases in order to develop three kinds of classification keys for participatory research projects. The first is concerning the application and combining of participatory tools, also regarding the methodological flow of interactions among social actors. The second classification key is associated with the territorial scales of approach and is dedicated to distinguish projects through their power to be allocated in a single scale or to transcend territories. The last is on the functionality of participatory processes since the objectives of social transformation can be distinctive without abandoning the perspective of fostering empowerment and learning through the production of hybrid knowledge.

5.2 Application of Participatory Tools

First of all, this classification is not merely as a try to associating quantity of participatory tools application or amount of collaborative working time with the quality of the dialogical intervention. Of course, the dedication in terms of a thoroughly ongoing process of subjects' engagement seems to be relevant to acquire a reasonable level of empowerment, social learning, and legitimate alternatives. However, considering that an excellent alternative to evaluate the process can be performed by understanding the results achieved (Kastelic et al. 2017; Oetzel et al. 2018), the amount of interactions is not necessarily converted into quality. Anyhow, the idea is to classify participatory approaches into three different categories considering the application of participatory tools: one-off, multi-tool, and cyclical approaches, see Table 5.1.

Even considering that, for instance, CBPR requires deep and legitimate engagement of social actors in all the research stages (Wallerstein et al. 2017), sometimes, interventions much more modest can deliver positive results. It is vital to recognize that social change, empowerment, and sustainability transitions with the engagement of vulnerable people are not easy to attain, but a participatory approach based just in a single participatory tool application can make some modest but distinguishable outcomes in comparison with regular qualitative investigations.

There are several differentiated experiences of participatory research with the application of just a unique tool, with no ongoing cyclical process. In the key classification by application of participatory tools, this kind of trial can be called a one-off approach. Of course, this type of initiative cannot be considered as a process of evolving engagement. Otherwise, it can enable responses in the sense of an

Table 5.1 Application of participatory tools to classify participatory approaches

Key	Characteristics
One-off	Initiatives where just one tool is applied; besides, not characterizing an ongoing process can provide embryonic dialogical interaction, reflection, and collaborative learning. Even being modest in terms of the challenges of participation, it can be differentiated for the generation of collaborative information, mainly in consideration of regular qualitative investigation like observation or application of interviews
Multi-tool	This is regarding combining participatory tools but not necessarily opening structure as to receive feedback from the subjects and to accept methodological changes alongside the process. It is very characteristic in projects with all the methodologies previously specified. Mainly, I consider this kind of application as a hesitation rooted in classical development of scientific research, where the researcher keeps with the intention of controlling the whole process. Although it seems to be not so legitimate in consideration of the essential assumptions of participatory research. There are many experiences in that way, and frequently they can provide some impressive results in terms of deepening understandings of socio-environmental and health determinants, besides promoting collaborative learning
Cyclical	Characterized by the successive application of participatory tools or collaborative research involving subjects as researchers. Feedbacks are essential concerning the ongoing methodological process of planning, acting, and fact finding. It allows critical participation on behalf of the subjects, and this is a central issue to legitimate the quality of the dialogical process as well as to enhance reciprocity and trust among different social actors involved. It means at sharing power with the subjects to empower them, meanwhile keeping the challenge of searching for the fundamental objectives of the project. The process characterizes itself as dynamic and adaptive (Lewin 1946; Toledo and Giatti 2014)

Source: elaborated by the author

embryonic dialogical interaction, and then it can provide in-depth explanations, fostering reflection and mutual learning at a certain level.

Nare et al. (2006) report an example of a one-off application of participatory tools in the realization of water quality monitoring and surveillance in Zimbabwe. Focus group as the applied participatory tool was associated with questionnaires, and the authors demonstrated the relevance to apprehend the local knowledge systems showing the perspective of integrating it with formal procedures of water quality monitoring systems.

Participatory research experience involved rural people in a region of pineapple monoculture in Costa Rica through the application of photovoice towards promoting collaborative ecosystem assessment, considering impoverished and resource-dependent communities (Berbés-Blázquez 2012). It is known that local knowledges and livelihoods' attributes are relevant to understand and act on the complexity of ecosystems services, and in that way, this one-off application could attain knowledge integration among diverse stakeholders and recognition of power imbalances. This experience reports to have catalyzed a contribution to communitarian empowerment and self-organization within the context of scarcity and the need to find synergies.

One-off application of participatory tools in this regard can provide good quality to deliver realistic expectations, and this type of rapid environmental or ecosystem services' appraisals can demonstrate that it is possible to reach distinct outcomes as desired in participatory research, and it occurs by the chosen on engaging subjects in the study. A participatory diagnosis can be more than a conventional one; the engagement of stakeholders provides cross-fertilization, cognitive inclusion, hybrid knowledge, and learning for both subjects and researchers. It also can provide some meta-information that could remain hidden in a diagnosis that just searches for environmental parameters and individual isolated perceptions and understandings.

The other two proposed categories, multi-tool and cyclical, have just one difference because both are associated with ongoing processes of applying multiple participatory tools in sequence. So, they are distinguishable because in cyclical approaches, it is necessary for sharing power through making good use of feedbacks that emerge in the ongoing process, and it must be related to the adaptive perspective of fact-finding and legitimate protagonism of the subjects to reshape the process. In other words, cyclical approaches must be friendly to changes and keen to the uncertainties in the development and redirections for methodological rounds. That is a relevant point in considering the quality of participatory processes on the criterion of trust and dialogical interaction, since multi-tool approaches, differently, are conceived rigidly and with no perspective for adaptive and self-organizing stance.

Multi-tool approaches are clearly recognizable by the characteristic of a preset static methodology, but even with no possibility to adaptations, they can provide results like social learning, reflection, and empowerment. Also, the nature of interaction can be of an excellent opportunity to produce several outcomes. However, the high level of participatory approach in consideration of the application of tools is cyclical, which can be genuinely symmetrical and can make possible a real integration of other cognitive contexts that should come with subjects' expectations, values, and mobilization to the targeted socio-environmental or post-normal problems. Actually, the cyclical approaches will be more complete in regard to incorporate uncertainties an ambiguity, those that must be progressively understood and considered in the negotiation for alternatives that balance risks and benefits. Such a perspective can be appropriate in mainstream frameworks of imbalanced power, knowledge possession, and vulnerabilities.

In a context of negligence and uncertain effects due to exposition of native indigenous communities to remnant nuclear radiation due to US weapons testing in the 1950s and 1960s, a participatory approach was dedicated to integrating subjects through researching on hazards in Nevada, Utah, and Southern California (USA). The approach involved full collaboration in all stages of the research, since the proposition of the project was acquiring and analyzing data, as well as interpreting data for publishing. The research activities focused on application of interviews, workshops, and technical research on contamination and health effects. The process of interaction allowed considering previous local knowledge and enabled local capacities for managing health risks, and eventually, it developed a community-based hazard management plan. Subjects were listened to and respected during the process, inducing adjustments in the activities—a relevant indicator of the cyclical approach. A collective critical sense emerged among the native communities, empowering them to dialog and participate in decision-making (Quigley et al. 2000).

The reported experience of ResNexus project in Guarulhos also gave some insights to understand the role of cyclical participatory approach by the relevance of local knowledge and wishes. In the implementation of the urban garden, diverse subjects were elementary for the entire duration of the project. They brought their particular previous farming backgrounds. Thus, it involved community dwellers, practitioners from the primary health care unit and from the local public school. The local collaborative knowledge on farming was built in meetings through the application of participatory tools and in the progress of collaborative working on the garden. All the decisions came through this process of new knowledge building, and it was fundamental to legitimate the dialogical approach and to allow that the involved social actors could appropriate the project.

Feedback from the process and from the subjects is key to characterize a cyclical participatory approach as to indicate a healthy ongoing and dialogical process of interaction. Essentially, this is not about the number of participatory tools applied. This is in regard to real engagement, sharing power, and a stance in which subjects understand that they have power to contribute in re-organizing the projects. When subjects realize their protagonism, it becomes natural to take action in operating new directions to the participatory process as well as to make real changes in their socio-ecological contexts. Cognitive inclusion raises in such a legitimate participatory process that changes itself when promoting changes in the context. This ecology of knowledge happens (Santos 2007) in cyclical and dialogical interactions, merging and resulting from an inexhaustible diversity, claiming from a perspective of indignation, and overcoming the hierarchy of knowledges.

5.3 Scales of Approach

The majority of experiences on participatory research projects dedicated to environmental and health issues can be characteristic of application on local scales, like in vulnerable communities, small villages, indigenous groups, social minorities, or specific risk groups as some professional categories (Giatti 2013, 2015). Even the adjective "community-based" makes sense of this tendency of local and small-scale approaches. Rescuing the inspiration from *Pedagogy of the Oppressed*, the circumstance of a local context in which education must be developed as an instrument of liberation from anti-dialogical actions is remarkable. However, in analogy, the oppressive processes are indeed being reproduced from larger scales, and with regard to unsustainability, determinants of health-related risks, and environmental injustices, all of these concerns manifesting locally but in hard association with cross-scale driving forces. Also, the burden of uncertainties and the causal chains of emergent and systemic threats have the same nature of crossing territorial scales.

That is a condition which is intensely reproduced in association with the success of modernity and the achievement of industrialization with the employment of new technologies. However, nowadays, we have witnessed the spillover of unexpected consequences that push forward local consequences as failures and emergent contradictions, generating a profusion of environmental degradation and risks. Locally, such processes can affect communities of marginalized and impoverished people, migrants, indigenous workers, and other easily understood as oppressed.

The challenge of the contemporary contexts of systemic interdependencies is to promote interactions among the local contexts with global scenarios and dynamics. Thus, a counterflow as bottom-up initiatives must be imperative to give recognition to local constraints and possibilities, finding responses capable of interacting with driven forces from upper scales. Local social practices and knowledges must encounter bridges and translations through cognitive inclusion that must be proficient at allowing dialogical interactions in which an action of a vulnerable person searching for survival encounters a conscious synergy with global concerns (Giatti et al. 2019). Those challenging relations between local and global scales are not merely a concern for marginalized and vulnerable people. The planetary awareness is a need for human development in a world of complexity in the face of emergent risks and uncertainties that can indistinctly affect the rich and poor in cross-temporal and spatial scales. Reflexivity is a vital issue for the contemporaneous society (Beck et al. 1995; Beck 2008), and participatory approaches are apparatuses to stimulating reflections involving plural social actors in different organizational levels, varied and contradictory stakes, and degrees of uncertainties. Participatory approaches must engender conditions to political protagonism for different social actors to deal with a political ecology that regularly ignores the diversity of societies, their own practices, and knowings, as well as their wishes, values, and cultures (Martínez Alier 2009; Leff 2017).

On these considerations, participatory approaches are distinguishable by the intended territorial scale of outreach. Moreover, the classification proposed in that way presents three key categories (see Table 5.2). The first one is "local," regarding the tendency of development of the mainstream experiences dealing with vulnerable social groups, and in a pertinent orientation, dedicating to reduce inequities, empowering people, and promoting change through engagement (Wallerstein et al. 2017). The second is called "expanded" and means at an upscaling process, like approaching broader territories through participation that many times require social representation. The last category and more sophisticated in terms of methodological design is "multilevel" and means at a transcendence within different scales.

In a systematic review of papers in Web of Science, searching for participatory research dedicated to environmental and health issues, among 170 experiences related to descriptive participatory methods and empiric data, 110 papers (64.7%) were on local approaches (Giatti 2013). For instance, a participatory approach held in agrarian communities in India, through participatory risk assessments, studied transitions on risk perceptions along decades. The interaction focused the local livelihood and the relation with transitions in environmental determinants that come from food insecurity and communicable diseases, to the make rise of contexts associated with globalization and late-modern world risk society (Jewitt and Baker 2012). Other examples for local approaches are easy to recognize like in communitarian diagnosis for health and environmental issues, and studies and interventions

Table 5.2 Territorial scales of intervention to classify participatory approaches

Key	Characteristics
Local	Refers to participatory approaches in which researchers usually have direct interactions with subjects of risks or some condition of inequity and socio-environmental vulnerability. The nomenclature "local" mainly indicates territorial identity of small groups like indigenous or riverine communities, slum dwellers, or other groups identified through cartographic attributes. Moreover, it can also refer to minorities like race and ethnicity, occupational groups, or risky behavioral groups
Expanded	Corresponds to upscaling approaches, like in cities, river basins, provinces, countries, or biomes. The participatory approach will be necessarily involving representatives of the socio diversity of the territorial cutting. Besides those social actors, it can also involve experts, decision-makers, and other public and private representatives. This territorial application is commonly associated with territorial planning, public policies, management of ecosystems, or decisions on the adoption of new technologies or chemical substances
Multilevel	This category is specifically on the challenging merging of local and expanded approaches, mainly in the direction of operating to legitimate the representativeness of local contexts to expanded territorial cuttings. Moreover, it must engage with feedback from expanded settings to local ones, since regularly, this kind of relation is unilateral with a predominance of prescriptive top-down stances. The main target is to make better arrangements and flows in the bottom-up sense. For targeting and constituting a counter-hegemonic movement, multilevel approaches are the most sophisticated in terms of promoting genuine dialogical interactions between social actors separated by abyssal differences like in terms of hegemonic knowledge and power appropriation

Source: elaborated by the author

involving peripheral urban communities in relation to their specific health inequities and respective contexts (Bisung et al. 2015; Belon et al. 2016; Berthold et al. 2017; Tucker et al. 2017).

In local approaches, the dialogical and reflexive processes have a significative relevance in terms of empowering people that many times can be inert without social capital to collective dealing with the dimensions of vulnerability. The proper interaction among subjects and researchers characterizes bridges to aggregate those vulnerable people from the isolation represented by social and cognitive exclusion. Accordingly, the process of local empowerment is related to the production of knowledges and respective appropriation, generating discourses, reports, or publications that gain remarkable representativeness in terms of advocacy. The process then assumes a feature of a corpus that can make dialogs hitherto impossible, opening pathways for major political intersections and perspectives to bring together communities, academics, and policymakers.

Expanded approaches, as presented in Table 4.2, can involve representatives in a broader territorial cutting in contrast with the small scale of local approaches. For example, in a province of Northern Vietnam on the Red River Delta, Hien et al. (2008) applied a participatory and intersectoral education process involving 150 communitarian leaders, focusing themes in healthy living environment promotion competency. In an urban scale, in Los Angeles/USA, participatory interventions on urban planning involved representatives of community-based nonprofit organizations in conceiving enigmatic urban spaces of alleys as possibilities of transitions into green infrastructures (Wolch et al. 2010). In regard to a broad agricultural area in Belgium, Wustenberghs et al. (2012) involved experts in setting up appropriate indicators targeting pesticide use and health impact assessment, targeting comprehensive chemical crop and farmers protection, in consideration of farmers' knowledge, awareness, and attitudes.

Increasing the potentialities of change in consideration of multiple causal chains and the need for integrated interventions, multilevel approaches must characterize dialogical processes within different scales. In that way, it is possible to verify such cross-scale interaction in an urban context, like related by Setti and Bógus (2010). It relates to implementation of Healthy Cities and Agenda 21 implementation in São Bernardo do Campo municipality, Brazil, and describes how public policy on the ecological neighborhood was developed by the involvement of 51 neighborhoods by collaborative work among citizens and policymakers to find measures to reduce environmental impacts and to recover water resources protected areas. Thus, this trial interplayed circumstances from the local dynamics interacting with the scale of municipal policymaking, also implied in the participatory process.

The legitimacy of a multilevel approach can take place since the outset of a local approach that through a political process encounters a proactive stance from a community to organize necessary scaling up interactions. That is called the bottom-up process, a remarkable accomplishment responding to the marginalization within socio-environmental vulnerability. For example, in a context of rapid socio-environmental changes in Nile Delta villages in Egypt, a participatory approach on schistosomiasis control involved local communities in prevention, subsequently engaging teachers, health workers and upscaling to the regional and national level of decision-making (Katsha and Watts 1997). Similarly, the case presented in Chap. 2 on the popular epidemiology empowering indigenous people in Ecuador in the face of oil contaminants and health risks also can be seen within a multilevel perspective since the social mobilization from local communities made protagonist in national law developments on oil exploitation (San Sebastián and Hurtig 2005).

Multilevel participatory approaches also can be a demand for dealing with disputes and bottlenecks that are challenging through different governance settings. Therefore, if participatory approaches can push forward integration of social actors into more democratic structures, disparities on power relations can also demand similar inclusion across distinct levels of governance. Within the European multilevel environmental governance, for instance, national governmental bodies can play less important roles. In that way, some Hungarian municipalities have shown various local impediments to deliver water supply according to the EU's directives, and it demonstrates the prevalence of top-down impositions causing governance failures, employing insufficient dealing with peripheral contexts (Leventon and Antypas 2012).

Considerations about territorial scales and participatory approaches can be appropriate to understand the challenge of change through the different contexts in necessary structural coupling with public policies, or even in the search for global governance on environmental and health-related issues. The complexity of post-normal problems reflects in part their conditionality to intertwined layers of stakes that involves social actors occasionally isolated by cognitive exclusion. Participatory approaches through multilevel interactions in that perspective must be a key initiative to overcome the most relevant rupture in the socio-ecological systems, since the ecology of knowledge can recover the self-organizing property of fostering bottom-up processes.

5.4 Functionality

This classification key is regarding the multiplicity of outcomes possibilities and the nature of the process as a product itself. Functionality can be understood as the quality of being functional and presenting a set of functions or capabilities associated with the process. The categories proposed (see Table 5.3) in this regard are conceived on the primordial objectives of the process in which the participatory project is designed. In this respect, the first category represents the participatory process simplified in terms of possible functions and restricted to a "diagnostic." The second category embodies the first and advances to a determination of promoting a change, and then it is named as "problem-solving." On the supposition of

Table 5.3 Functionality to classify participatory approaches

Key	Characteristics
Diagnostic	Limits itself to participatory recognition of a problem or a context. Generally is developed through an interdisciplinary framework as having obligatory recognition of the nature of common sense to interact with different areas of knowledge. Beyond regular basic diagnostics, by the premise of involving stakeholders, it favors encompassing richness in terms of qualitative information (like meta-information) and production of hybrid knowledge, fostering social learning
Problem-solving	Collaborative searching alternatives for complex problems, demanding previous diagnosis, and ongoing reflections. Also concerns to associate capacities from the different social actors involved in the process, as well as to find possible resources and partnerships that can contribute to the strategies to promote concrete change in socio-ecological systems. Empowerment and dialogical interactions belong to the ongoing development of activities and play a vital role in the perspective of change
Post-normal problems	Uncertainties and emergent systems' risks must be crucial questions in the dialogical process. The involvement of social actors is fundamental to encourage critical control on decisions towards complex issues permeated by insufficient awareness of possible unfolding and emergent systemic properties. Besides involving diagnostics and problem-solving stances, post-normal problems require pushing forward more democratic structures of governance to deliver socially robust scientific knowledge and decision-making

Source: elaborated by the author

evolving though increasing in functions, the third and maybe a more ambitious category is to target "post-normal problems." In that direction, this last category can embody both diagnostics and problem-solving, but the primary concern of its legitimacy must be on the perspective of dealing with problems involving different social actors and embracing uncertainties and possible values in dispute alongside the dialogical development.

Besides making a simple diagnostic, this first level of functionality in participatory approaches also must represent social and cognitive inclusion and it can also promote the dynamic duality of teaching–learning for both subjects and researchers. Therefore, it makes much more sense than just diagnosing, playing an essential role in democratizing knowledge. For instance, Stern et al. (2010) describe participatory research held in Cape Town periphery, South Africa, in which risk factors on non-communicable diseases are collaboratively studied searching for better understanding on the role of the interplay of socio-environmental and behavioral practices. As the diagnosis becomes appropriated by the involved communities, strengthening of social capital happens to promote engagement and health.

In a search for better farming productivity and sustainability through practices of irrigation in a scenario of scarcity and fragmented governance of water resources in Tunisia, Hanafi et al. (2018) present the power of participation in a shared diagnosis by application of focus groups and meetings. In comparison with a preview application of single interviews, the authors show that a participatory approach can unveil power relations and the need for collective understanding and action on the complex and conflicting issue of using the common water resource. This case also shows that the limits of participatory diagnosis can be overlapping on the need for building problem-solving alternatives. The rise of social mobilization in the process induces reflection and a flow of understandings and dialogs that conduct the social actors in finding collaborative solutions. Consequently, better than considering the relevance of primal objectives of a participatory approach, it is more relevant to facilitate and to allow the self-organizing process through legitimate engagement. This autopoietic feature can result in a myriad of outcomes, bringing more insights, alternatives, actions, and knowledges than previously conceived by the researchers.

When the functionality of a participatory approach moves forward to higher levels of complexities and uncertainties, there is a possible analogy with post-normal problems and their background in terms of dichotomies of facts and values, misunderstandings on knowledge and ignorance, high stakes, and the need for immediate actions on unknown emergent and systemic problems (Funtowicz and Ravetz 1993).

Either by self-organizing processes or by previously established procedures, participatory processes embracing post-normal problems concerns to a kind of empowerment that allows a layperson with common sense find pathways for dialog with high-complexity issues, experts, and decision-makers. To be specific, this is a procedure to make a critical control on the production of knowledge on ambivalent and uncertain issues and respective decision-making. It is not in defense of an anti-science stance; these kinds of dialogical interactions must operate in the intersection area of high stakes and high uncertainties, where the merit of decision must be reflexive, considering benefits, conflicts of interest, and also the costs for precaution. For example, in the way of considering what should be losses in terms of refusing a new technology, and what if it brings unknown and dangerous possibilities. Therefore, it is much more on taking conscious and multi-stakeholder decisions than in just adopting one or another scientific discourse. Remember that scientific paradigms can live side by side even when presenting antagonisms (Kuhn 1992), and the academic world can be permeated by policy (Van den Hove 2007).

Global climate change and possible consequences are very emblematic in that way. Beyond political and cultural background on the relevance of this planetary issue (Hoffman 2015), it is time to bring society to work together in different forms of organization and levels of governance to stimulate and create alternatives for mitigation and adaptation. Also, it is time to rescue the possibilities of merging local knowledge and social practices with multi-scale engagements to make possible what is really needed: different solutions and possibilities for different contexts, building resiliences from local to global.

Berkes and Berkes (2009) relate the participation of Canadian indigenous in a study that encompasses climate change abnormalities associated with other environmental constraints. The characteristic holism of native people and continued reading of the environment provide the basis for knowledge production. In that direction, the intervention proposed considered availability and management of natural resources within uncertain scenarios through collective mental models able to adjust to new information; in other words, an adaptive framework.

Also committed to climate change, but in urban peripheral contexts in Brazil, Trajber et al. (2019) show the relevance of a looping methodology to interplay with youth agency possibilities of learning in an action research project. The intervention targeted disaster risk reduction. Through dialogical interactions this project raised emergent insights and action-oriented collaborative agendas, outperforming local and scientific isolated capacities.

In the perspective of precaution with the high speed of technological innovations, another post-normal problem frame can be associated with the use of nanotechnologies. As a multi-stakeholder participatory process to envisage related risks and stakes, Wiek et al. (2009) report systemic scenario planning involving multiple stakeholders in Switzerland promoted reflections on the employment of nanotechnologies in five different scenarios, stimulating perceptions, highlighting the need for more integrated governance, recognition of social amplification of risks, and the stance of public awareness, consumption, and risk tolerance. Accordingly, scenario planning has been a good exercise for involving multiple stakeholders in a process of social learning and choosing alternatives for better futures considering variables that are currently decisive. Furthermore, it has been applied with good efficiency to bring social actors and institutions to plan and act in better public policies (Peterson et al. 2003; Godet and Durance 2009).

5.5 Understanding the Plurality of Participatory Approaches

The frontiers of the categories presented in this taxonomy are not rigid, since the most important thing is to recognize diversity and possibility of applications and the search for the joining target of researching as intervening and vice versa. Anyhow, it is essential to remark that all three classifications proposed can be seen in the sense of evolving processes within complex demands. In that direction from a one-off application to a cyclical one, there is the pathway of developing a dialogical process to increase possible and diverse outcomes. The interplay from a local to a multilevel approach also sounds to extend the possibilities; it makes the commendable interaction with multi-scale determinants and fosters the opportunity to deal with public policies and more democratic governance structures. Also, in a precise sequential evolution, a participatory process can become more sophisticated in consideration of the contemporary socio-ecological and health issues when it begins with a diagnosis, evolves into the search of collaborative actions and problem-solving, and finally reaches the frame of embracing uncertainties.

The incorporation of climate change-related issues and uncertainties can be a synthesis of this possible evolution through classes and categories of participatory research. It can occur as connecting local dynamics, constraints, social practices, and knowledges through different scales. Even the collaboration with academics plays a role in this procedure, also advocating possible coupling with knowledges and practices at the level of local public decision-making, then to other interlocutions and governance levels. The approaching of a post-normal issue like climate change also makes imperative cyclical approaches as so to qualify a high dialogical level in terms of participatory research, delivering relevant reflection, recognition of uncertainties, and values in dispute.

In regard to the related experience of action research in Iauaretê (Toledo et al. 2012; Toledo and Giatti 2014), the indigenous community in Amazon, Brazil, the participatory process began as a local approach designed to be cyclical. The evolving process showed the need to interact with policy makers since there was a severe lack of infrastructure that would only be possible with public investments. Also, the same precarious sanitary conditions of Iauaretê were reproduced in tens of similar communities in the same region. From the interactive process with the community, the understanding was to promote advocacy within the inertia of decision-makers to improve water, sanitation, and other preventive health benefits. This proactive stance emerged from the dialogical process itself, as a product, as a new understanding, and also, in the form of new co-created empirical evidence.

Again, the amount of participatory tools or the perspective of evolving through the proposed categories is not a signal of quality. However, the understanding of this point of view in which participatory processes are plural, "alive," and self-organizing can contribute for better planning and managing of such projects and respective diversity of outcomes. The decision on conducting participatory research as mentioned before has a political dimension, and its effects are transforming subjects and researchers through symmetrical and dynamical relationships and actions in the concrete world. The recognition of classes and categories of transitions in that way can help in better assessment of and response to feedbacks of the process.

References

Beck, U. (2008). *La Sociedade del Riesgo Mundial: em busca de la seguridade*. Barcelona: Paidós.

Beck, U., Giddens, A., & Lash, S. (1995). *Modernização reflexiva*. São Paulo: Unesp.

Belon, A. P., Nieuwendyk, L. M., Vallianatos, H., & Nykiforuk, C. I. (2016). Community lenses revealing the role of sociocultural environment on physical activity. *American Journal of Health Promotion, 30*, e92–e100.

Berbés-Blázquez, M. (2012). A participatory assessment of ecosystem services and human wellbeing in rural Costa Rica using photo-voice. *Environmental Management, 49*, 862–875.

Berkes, F., & Berkes, M. K. (2009). Ecological complexity, fuzzy logic, and holism in indigenous knowledge. *Futures, 41*, 6–12. https://doi.org/10.1016/j.futures.2008.07.003.

Berthold, S. M., Kong, S., Kuoch, T., et al. (2017). Combating health disparities in Cambodian American communities: A CBPR approach to building community capacity. *Progress in Community Health Partnerships: Research, Education, and Action, 11*, 109–118.

Bisung, E., Elliott, S. J., Abudho, B., et al. (2015). Using photovoice as a community based participatory research tool for changing water, sanitation, and hygiene behaviours in Usoma, Kenya. *BioMed Research International, 2015*, 903025.

Brydon-Miller, M., Greenwood, D., & Maguire, P. (2003). *Why action research?* London: Sage Publications.

Funtowicz, S. O., & Ravetz, J. R. (1993). Science for the post-normal age. *Futures, 25*, 739–755.

Giatti, L. L. (2013). *Uma contribuição à Ciência pós-normal: aplicações e desafios da ampliação da comunidade de pares em contextos socioambientais e de saúde*. PhD Thesis, Universidade de São Paulo.

Giatti, L. L. (2015). *O paradigma da ciência pós normal: participação social na produção de saberes e na governança socioambiental e da saúde*. São Paulo: Annablume.

Giatti, L. L., Urbinatti, A. M., & Carvalho, C. M., et al. (2019-ahead to print). *Nexos de exclusão e desafios de sustentabilidade e saúde em uma periferia urbana*. Cadernos de Saude Publica.

Godet, M., & Durance, P. (2009). *La prospectiva estratégica*. Paris: Lipsor.

Hanafi, S., Marlet, S., Jamin, J.-Y., et al. (2018). Participation in a complex and conflicting context: Implementing a shared diagnosis in a Northern Tunisia irrigation scheme. *Irrigation and Drainage*.

Hien, L. T. T., Takano, T., Seino, K., et al. (2008). Effectiveness of a capacity-building program for community leaders in a healthy living environment: A randomized community-based intervention in rural Vietnam. *Health Promotion International, 23*, 354–364.

Hoffman, A. J. (2015). *How culture shapes the climate change debate*. Palo Alto, CA: Stanford University Press.

Jewitt, S., & Baker, K. (2012). Risk, wealth and agrarian change in India. Household-level hazards vs. late-modern global risks at different points along the risk transition. *Global Environmental Change, 22*, 547–557.

Kastelic, S. L., Wallerstein, N., Duran, B., & Oetzel, J. G. (2017). Socio-ecologic framework for CBPR. In *Community-based participatory research for health: Advancing social and health equity* (p. 77).

Katsha, S., & Watts, S. (1997). Schistosomiasis in two Nile delta villages: An anthropological perspective. *Tropical Medicine & International Health, 2*, 846–854.

Kuhn, T. A. (1992). *A estrutura das revoluções científicas*. São Paulo: Perspectiva.

Leff, E. (2017). Power-knowledge relations in the field of political ecology. *Ambiente and Sociedade, 20*, 225–256.
Leventon, J., & Antypas, A. (2012). Multi-level governance, multi-level deficits: The case of drinking water management in Hungary. *Environmental Policy and Governance, 22*, 253–267.
Lewin, K. (1946). Action research and minority problems. *Journal of Social Issues, 2*, 34–46.
Martínez Alier, J. (2009). O ecologismo dos pobres: conflitos ambientais e linguagens de valoração. In *O ecologismo dos pobres: conflitos ambientais e linguagens de valoração* (p. 379).
Nare, L., Love, D., & Hoko, Z. (2006). Involvement of stakeholders in the water quality monitoring and surveillance system: The case of Mzingwane catchment, Zimbabwe. *Physics and Chemistry of the Earth, Parts A/B/C, 31*, 707–712.
Oetzel, J. G., Wallerstein, N., Duran, B., et al. (2018). Impact of participatory health research: A test of the community-based participatory research conceptual model. *BioMed Research International, 2018*, 7281405.
Peterson, G. D., Cumming, G. S., & Carpenter, S. R. (2003). Scenario planning: A tool for conservation in an uncertain world. *Conservation Biology, 17*, 358–366.
Quigley, D., Sanchez, V., Handy, D., et al. (2000). Participatory research strategies in nuclear risk management for native communities. *Journal of Health Communication, 5*, 305–331.
San Sebastián, M., & Hurtig, A. K. (2005). Oil development and health in the Amazon basin of Ecuador: The popular epidemiology process. *Social Science & Medicine, 60*, 799–807.
Santos, B. S. (2007). Para além do pensamento abissal: das linhas globais a uma ecologia de saberes. *Novos estudos-CEBRAP*, 71–94.
Setti, A. F. F., & Bógus, C. M. (2010). Community participation in an intervention program developed in a protected area. *Saude e Sociedade, 19*, 946–960.
Stern, R., Puoane, T., & Tsolekile, L. (2010). Peer reviewed: An exploration into the determinants of noncommunicable diseases among rural-to-urban migrants in Periurban South Africa. *Preventing Chronic Disease, 7*, A131.
Toledo, R. F., & Giatti, L. L. (2014). Challenges to participation in action research. *Health Promotion International, 30*, 162–173.
Toledo, R. F. d., Giatti, L. L., & Pelicioni, M. C. F. (2012). Social mobilization in health and sanitation in an action research process in an indigenous community in northwestern amazon. *Saúde e Sociedade, 21*, 206–218.
Trajber, R., Walker, C., Marchezini, V., et al. (2019). Promoting climate change transformation with young people in Brazil: Participatory action research through a looping approach. *Action Research, 17*, 87–107.
Tucker, C. M., Wippold, G. M., Williams, J. L., et al. (2017). A CBPR study to test the impact of a church-based health empowerment program on health behaviors and health outcomes of black adult churchgoers. *Journal of Racial and Ethnic Health Disparities, 4*, 70–78.
Van den Hove, S. (2007). A rationale for science–policy interfaces. *Futures, 39*, 807–826.
Wallerstein, N., Duran, B., Minkler, M., & Oetzel, J. G. (2017). *Community-based participatory research for health: Advancing social and health equity*. Hoboken, NJ: Wiley.
Wiek, A., Gasser, L., & Siegrist, M. (2009). Systemic scenarios of nanotechnology: Sustainable governance of emerging technologies. *Futures, 41*, 284–300.
Wolch, J., Newell, J., Seymour, M., et al. (2010). The forgotten and the future: Reclaiming back alleys for a sustainable city. *Environment and Planning A, 42*, 2874–2896.
Wustenberghs, H., Delcour, I., D'haene, K., et al. (2012). A dual indicator set to help farms achieve more sustainable crop protection. *Pest Management Science, 68*, 1130–1140.

Chapter 6
Concluding on the Role of Participatory Approaches in Post-Normal Times

> *Then we waited. We rested our rifles for a while, without firing a single shot. We wanted to give them a truce during which to finish of our poor ponies. Even after the last whimper had died on the air, we remained appalled and quiet for a long time, until the sounds and the silence, and the remembrance of that suffering should begin to recede in the distance. After that, everything started up all over again, even more fiercely. And in what I am telling, we see the desolation of the world. God exists, yes, slowly and suddenly. He acts, all right—but almost wholly through the medium of persons, good and bad. The awesome things of this world! The backlands are a powerful weapon. Is God a trigger?*
>
> *João Guimarães Rosa (From the book "The Devil to Pay in the Backlands"—(Guimarães Rosa 1963). In this prominent and thrilling novel, Riobaldo Tatarana, a gunman fighting in the backlands, raises universal existential questions from his context, and so, making philosophical connections of his distant wilderness with the world).*

There is too much beauty in worlds' diversity, so the diversity of societies and their knowledges are not only splendid but also fundamental pieces in the completeness of socio-ecological systems on the global scale. On the one hand, local culture and knowledge can have peculiar ways of translating and understanding cross-scale and global problems into communitarian dynamics. On the other hand, such cultural and epistemic uniqueness is crucial for finding alternatives for global concerns to encounter accession and viability into local scales. Moreover, local culture is a key element to interact and dialog with the burden of uncertainties and possible consequences of decision-making on scientific assumptions.

There is no perspective for sustainability without promoting interactions towards these scales and detached collectives and institutions. It remains to exist abyssal inconsistencies in terms of power, capacities, and possession of hegemonic knowledge, and this is something to inhibit intended coupling diversities and ecology of knowledge (Santos 2009). An expressive obstruction for interaction among different social actors seems to be the cognitive exclusion. Beyond the insufficient interactions

L. L. Giatti, *Participatory Research in the Post-Normal Age*,
https://doi.org/10.1007/978-3-030-27924-0_6

and asymmetrical relationships, alienation of large amounts of people represents a severe concern about political decisions to be made on questions that exceed the limits of scientific certainty. The interplay of unsustainability complexities, emergent and systemic risks, scientific uncertainties, high stakes, and controversies in values has shaped new forms of oppression, new faces of oppressors, and demands for innovative practices to knowledge production and respective applicability.

To build new alternatives on the contemporary crisis, some concepts on Paulo Freire's pedagogy (Freire 2000) can contribute to the reflexive search for innovative pathways. Among those concepts are: dividing to rule; manipulation; cooperation; and organization.

The current contexts of oppression also consists of segregating, and then the abyssal lines of cognitive exclusion seem to be aligned to the perspective of dividing to rule. The more advanced scientific discourses become, the farther they are from common sense. The marginalization of nonacademic knowledge also contributes to segregate social groups far from decision-making and political protagonism. The extent of such ruptures can even be related to disasters of cognitive exclusion, where anti-dialogical actions entail in the causality and in the amplification of consequences.

When a technological disaster occurs, exhibiting previous negligence of uncertainties and scientific limits, those affected and previously alienated from controlling the quality of decisions realize themselves as their own oppressors. In such a scenario, oppressed as oppressors can just play the game for the social actors that had power and benefit from the decisions taken on high stakes, with a lack of transparency or even negligence. For instance, the offer of a new technology to create new needs meanwhile turning a blind eye to possible emergent and systemic risks can represent a false generosity.

Otherwise, lack of deepening and participatory interactions can matter when a relatively well-resolved scientific question is treated without considering other layers of intertwined determinants. For example, sanitary measures cannot achieve objectives of health promotion when socio-cultural backgrounds (i.e., sanitation in indigenous lands with the local mythical conditionings) are not considered. Such background would require social mobilization, empowerment, and collaborative learning and action.

All of these ruptures can be associated with anti-dialogical postures, and so maintaining a context of fragmentation on one side, and in another dispossession and domain on power and knowledge. Manipulation also serves to this end, and this can be operated through propaganda, mass communication, inducement of myths, and the subjugation of people with the marginalization of nonacademic knowledge. The anti-dialogical reproduction is an indispensable requisite to keep the status quo, and so cognitive exclusion plays a to our convenience, even when we realize processes that target social inclusion with no consideration of the compelling apprehension of the cognitive field.

Then, these ongoing manipulation processes often disregard communities as a whole and something belonging to a dimension of a totality. In that way, there is an imperative of conceiving the holarchic structures (systems inside other systems) through the dialogical cognitive interactions among scales into the wholeness. That is the appeal for possible bottom-up interactions in consideration of local knowledges and practices, instead of the dominant top-down prescriptive and oppressive actions.

To acknowledge potentialities from the local contexts or communities, cooperation and organization must be realized as foundational capabilities, as well as determinants of the success or failure for any intervention. Both characteristics are requirements in dialogical interactions and represent to assume people's strengths to legitimate democratic structures, also in considering the need for better governance structures to involve diverse stakeholders on environmental resources constraints, for example.

Organization is antagonistic to anti-dialogical action and manipulation (see Fig. 6.1). Thus, since the individual level, organization represents collectives to act together, playing a dialectic between the sub and superstructures. The pedagogy of participatory research approaches can rescue and reinforce such capacity. The ongoing unpacking of generative themes anchored in the local reality, as well as the moving on coding and decoding situations, are significant in the possibility of local people to reach and interact with issues, languages, and social actors in other never-before-reachable levels. Organization is inherent of human beings in their personal capabilities, enabling the power to act on the real world as the ongoing process of

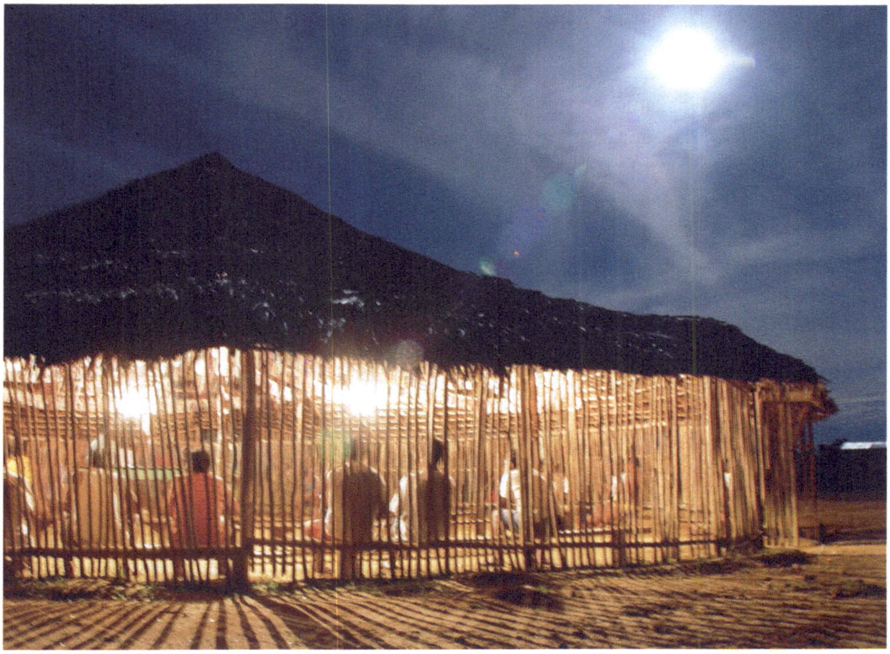

Fig. 6.1 A regular meeting in a community center in Iauaretê, Brazilian Amazon. Organization and collective conversation is inherent to the indigenous culture. Source: the author

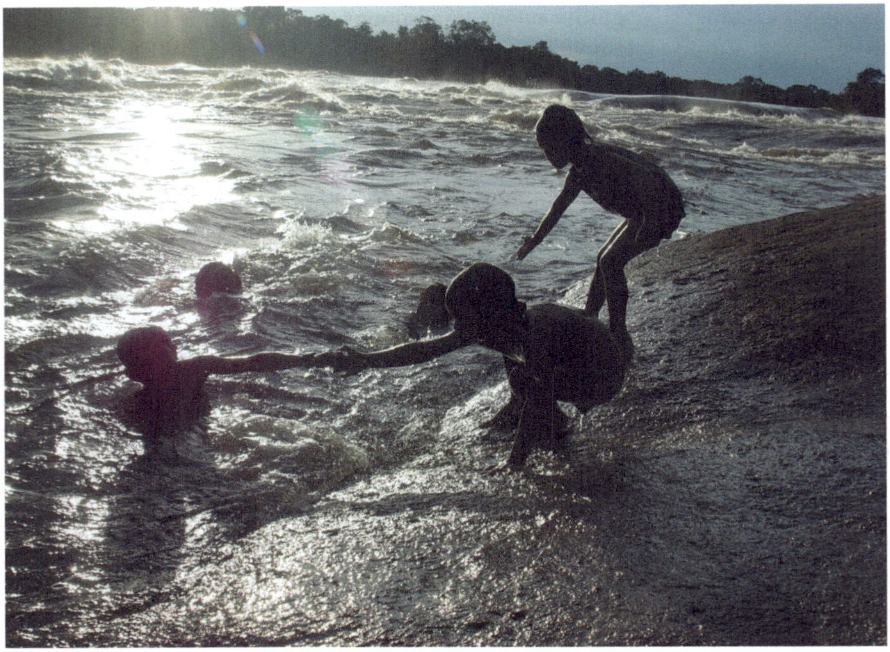

Fig. 6.2 Cooperation is natural among humans, and it is a component of our self-organizing capabilities. Source: the author

changing themselves, that is, the property of autonomy and autopoiesis (Maturana and Varela 1992). Cooperation, as well, is another inherent capability (see Fig. 6.2), in which subjects can burst domination through action on transforming the world. The evolution of cooperative associations of humans, communities, and institutions can be a different look and an alternative to the exacerbated contemporary competitiveness. In regard of the current complex issues, cooperation appears to be relevant through enhancing local capacities and joining partnerships of distinct social actors and institutions, extending conjunction with capacities outside of the local context (Wallerstein et al. 2017).

Participatory research plays a considerable amount of possibilities for dialogical interaction, fostering organization, cooperation, and coupling in the sense of ecologizing knowledges and capabilities. The procedure of building possible interaction of distinct social actors enables to promote actions as a cultural synthesis. Also, this synthesis becomes practicable even as encompassing knowledges that have been marginalized, but on the other hand, considering such knowledges as crucial for engaging people and finding robust solutions to the complex current issues. In participatory approaches, there is the perspective of making a parallel of actions and interactions. Intersubjectivity, trust, sharing power, and legitimate reciprocity provide a symmetrical interaction, and in such a ground it is possible to associate different social actors' mobilization into a convergent action.

Besides, the process of participatory research itself brings much more possibilities and generates a diversity of outputs, insights, understandings, and innovation. The strengthening of the self-organizing property of a collective transcends the conventional production of scientific investigation and so outperforms initial expectations for intervention over a real problem. In the production of information and knowledge, that can be used by researchers and by the subjects, participatory processes produce intrinsic, dynamic, and reflexive benefits, like meta-information, that can embrace relevant explanations of unknown factors. In the process of intervening through actions, the same, the ongoing dialogical process gains new directions on new collective understandings, and so innovative possibilities. This creative feature and the respective diversity of doings and knowings can entail scenarios of more sustainability, increasing adaptive capacity, and then elevating the resilience of a socio-ecological system to disturbances, like those associated with consequences of climate change.

For those post-normal problems, with high stakes and uncertainties, the participatory processes, by the premise of sharing power and having an adaptive methodology, facilitate integrating uncertainties in reflexive interactions among subjects. Accordingly, different stakes and possible risks can be put in collective multi-stakeholder reflection, also helping to frame socially robust scientific knowledge (Gibbons 1999).

In this regard, the question is not only promoting that laypersons have means of appropriating scientific culture. More than this, the relationship of science, the appliance of science, and a broader societal involvement must constitute the milieu for dialogical interactions. That stance relates to a perspective to contributing to reducing a big gap, collaborating to real translations among different cognitive frames, and so achieving fairer social inclusion on the perspective of ecology of knowledge.

Participatory research will never be better than traditional objective and specialized scientific production. Indeed, there is no competition in that way. Dialogical interactions as a search for involving stakeholders in the research process are, in fact, a perspective of making a critical control on how science is to be applied, considering the limits of scientific production, antagonisms on paradigms, ambiguity, stakes, and risks to the participants. Extended peer communities can become an objective to be pursued with the adoption of participatory methodologies. In addition, the frame of critical control must reinforce the applicability of excellent quality of scientific production, helping people to avoid anti-science postures and consequences, like in the worrying vaccination mistrust.

Understanding multiple possibilities and features of adaptive participatory approaches also can give support to better choices and outreach of projects in terms of collaborative production of knowledge, empowerment, and interventions. For that, the three classification keys present a framework to apprehend such diversity in terms of the application of participatory tools, in the relation of scales of approach, and also in the varied functionalities for such projects. That is an effort to help planning participatory research, but also a background to correlate alternatives with the realization of satisfactory scientific evidence and learning, besides tangible actions.

In this classificatory proposal, it is understood that cyclical multilevel approaches with the possibility of integrating uncertainties can characterize alternatives to reach correspondence to post-normal problems. In that way, the contemporary challenges of sustainability in the face of global–local interfaces, the multiplicity of driven forces in a complex chain with the inherent unpredictability can be matching with this kind of sophisticated ongoing trials.

Also, considering the contemporary post-normal, a new theory of revolutionary action must engage with such complexities, uncertainties, and levels of demanded responses. On Freirian assumption, we are incomplete beings, our societies are incomplete in the context of the rapid evolution of technological innovation associated with growing and interdependent global scarcities. For that, our constant challenge must be ongoing in dialogical interactions, overlapping barriers, reducing inequities and social exclusion, and enhancing our humanistic features into democratic structures of collaborative learning and researching.

References

Freire, P. (2000). *Pedagogy of the oppressed* (30th anniversary ed.). (M. B. Ramos, Trans., D. Macedo, Intro.). New York City: The Continuum International Publishing Group.

Gibbons, M. (1999). Science's new social contract with society. *Nature, 402*, C81.

Guimarães Rosa, J. (1963). *The devil to pay in the backlands*. (J. L. Taylor and H. de Onis, Trans.) New York: Knopf.

Maturana, H. R., & Varela, F. J. (1992). *The tree of knowledge* (rev. ed.). Boston: Shambala.

Santos, B. S. (2009). *Una epistemología del sur: la reinvención del conocimiento y la emancipación social*. Siglo XXI.

Wallerstein, N., Duran, B., Minkler, M., & Oetzel, J. G. (2017). *Community-based participatory research for health: Advancing social and health equity*. Hoboken, NJ: Wiley.

Index

L. L. Giatti, *Participatory Research in the Post-Normal Age*,
https://doi.org/10.1007/978-3-030-27924-0

D

E

The manufacturer's authorised representative in the EU is Springer
Nature Customer Service Centre GmbH, Europaplatz 3, 69115 Heidelberg,
Germany. If you have any concerns regarding our products, please
contact ProductSafety@springernature.com

Printed and bound by CPI Group (UK) Ltd, Croydon, CR0 4YY
05/10/2026
02228156-0002